Advances in Experimental Medicine and Biology

Volume 1242

Series Editors

Advances in Experimental Medicine and Biology provides a platform for scientific contributions in the main disciplines of the biomedicine and the life sciences. This series publishes thematic volumes on contemporary research in the areas of microbiology, immunology, neurosciences, biochemistry, biomedical engineering, genetics, physiology, and cancer research. Covering emerging topics and techniques in basic and clinical science, it brings together clinicians and researchers from various fields.

Advances in Experimental Medicine and Biology has been publishing exceptional works in the field for over 40 years, and is indexed in SCOPUS, Medline (PubMed), Journal Citation Reports/Science Edition, Science Citation Index Expanded (SciSearch, Web of Science), EMBASE, BIOSIS, Reaxys, EMBiology, the Chemical Abstracts Service (CAS), and Pathway Studio.

2018 Impact Factor: 2.126.

More information about this series at http://www.springer.com/series/5584

Liane Deligdisch-Schor • Angelica Mareş Miceli
Editors

Hormonal Pathology of the Uterus

Springer

Editors
Liane Deligdisch-Schor
Professor Emeritus
Department of Pathology
Icahn School of Medicine at Mount Sinai
New York, NY, USA

Department of Obstetrics-Gynecology
and Reproductive Science
Icahn School of Medicine at Mount Sinai
New York, NY, USA

Angelica Mareş Miceli
New York Medical College
Westchester Medical Center
Valhalla, NY, USA

ISSN 0065-2598 ISSN 2214-8019 (electronic)
Advances in Experimental Medicine and Biology
ISBN 978-3-030-38476-0 ISBN 978-3-030-38474-6 (eBook)
https://doi.org/10.1007/978-3-030-38474-6

This Springer imprint is published by the registered company Springer Nature Switzerland AG
The registered company address is: Gewerbestrasse 11, 6330 Cham, Switzerland

Contents

Contributors

David Barad Mt Sinai West, New York, NY, USA

Center for Human Reproduction (CHR), New York, NY, USA

Liane Deligdisch-Schor Professor Emeritus, Department of Pathology, Icahn School of Medicine at Mount Sinai, New York, NY, USA

Department of Obstetrics-Gynecology and Reproductive Science, Icahn School of Medicine at Mount Sinai, New York, NY, USA

Pouya Javadian Robert Wood Johnson Barnabas Health Newark Beth Israel Medical Center, Newark, NJ, USA

Myriam Kossaï Department of Pathology and Molecular Pathology, Centre Jean Perrin, Clermont-Ferrand, France

UMR INSERM 1240, Universite Clermont Auvergne, Clermont-Ferrand, France

Angelica Mareş Miceli New York Medical College, Westchester Medical Center, Valhalla, NY, USA

Farr R. Nezhat Nezhat Surgery for Gynecology/Oncology, New York, NY, USA

Weill Cornell Medical College of Cornell University, New York, NY, USA

Stony Brook University School of Medicine, Stony Brook, NY, USA

Department of Minimally Invasive Gynecologic Surgery and Robotics, NYU Winthrop University Hospital, Mineola, NY, USA

John Paciuc Lenox Hill Hospital, Mount Sinai Hospital, New York, NY, USA

Tanja Pejovic Department of ObGyn, Oregon Health and Science University, Portland, OR, USA

Frédérique Penault-Llorca Department of Pathology and Molecular Pathology, Centre Jean Perrin, Clermont-Ferrand, France

UMR INSERM 1240, Universite Clermont Auvergne, Clermont-Ferrand, France

Sarah Thisted University of British Columbia, Vancouver, BC, Canada

Michael White Department of Minimally Invasive Gynecologic Surgery, NYU-Winthrop University Hospital, Mineola, NY, USA

Hormonal Biophysiology of the Uterus

Liane Deligdisch-Schor and Angelica Mareş Miceli

1 Uterine Development

The uterus is derived from the fusion of Müllerian ducts originating from the mesodermal genital ridge, starting at their caudal end and progressing up. This event starts in the invagination of coelomic epithelium, around the sixth week in utero (i.u.). Cervical glands appear by 15 weeks and endometrial glands as well as myometrial tissue around 19 weeks i.u. This development occurs under the influence of the maternal steroid sex hormones circulating from the maternal blood via the placenta into the fetal circulation. Müllerian duct development is normally inhibited in the male fetus by androgens and by a nonsteroidal hormone, Müllerian inhibiting substance (MIS) produced by the Sertoli cells of the testis [1, 2]. Congenital anomalies of the uterus are rare, mostly resulting from imperfect or absent fusion of the Müllerian ducts or atresia associated with an autosomal recessive or dominant genetic defect.

The endometrium at birth is usually at resting phase, inactive, and consists of a single layer of cuboidal epithelium with sparse glands surrounded by spindle-shaped stromal cells. Maternal hormonal influence however may elicit proliferative and secretory changes due to estrogenic and progesterone activity and even predecidual changes during intrauterine life with rare menstrual changes in the neonate. After delivery the endometrium normally reverts to its resting phase until menarche.

L. Deligdisch-Schor (✉)
Professor Emeritus, Department of Pathology, Icahn School of Medicine at Mount Sinai, New York, NY, USA

Department of Obstetrics-Gynecology and Reproductive Science, Icahn School of Medicine at Mount Sinai, New York, NY, USA
e-mail: Liane.deligdisch@mssm.edu

A. Mareş Miceli
New York Medical College, Westchester Medical Center, Valhalla, NY, USA
e-mail: amares@nymc.edu

L. Deligdisch-Schor, A. Mareş Miceli (eds.), *Hormonal Pathology of the Uterus*, Advances in Experimental Medicine and Biology 1242,
https://doi.org/10.1007/978-3-030-38474-6_1

The GnRH pulse generator is capable to induce ovarian follicle maturation and estrogen synthesis and secretion during intrauterine development of the female fetus and resumes this activity with the advent of menarche. At birth, with the acute loss of placental and maternal hormones, the neonate hypothalamus-placental-ovary system is released from negative suppression. It resumes secretion of GnRH stimulation and FSH and LH release for about the first 6 months of life, after which this secretion declines. Leptin, a substance produced in the adipocytes, plays an important role having the ability to activate the central elements controlling the hypothalamic pulse generator and the onset of puberty.

Puberty starts with nocturnal pulses of gonadotropin secretion with LH exceeding FSH, generating increase in serum estradiol which increments LH secretion by the anterior pituitary resulting later in full secretion of gonadotropins.

After a decade of quiescence, GnRH pulsatile secretion resumes at daytime, and gradually repetitive ovulatory cycles emerge. The ovarian steroid hormone secretion elicits a maturation process of the uterus: the corpus uteri grows first faster than the cervix, and the endometrium matures with established cycles of proliferation, secretion, and menstrual shedding following the cyclic stimulation and withdrawal feedback mechanisms of the pituitary-ovarian system.

Menarche usually occurs between 9 and 16 years of age, after secondary sexual characteristics have begun their development. The first menstrual cycles are usually non-ovulatory and irregular, with intervals of 2–3 months. Once regularly established the cycles last 3–6 weeks, with menstrual shedding occurring 2 weeks after ovulation. The preovulatory phase is variable, while the postovulatory phase is relatively constant. The menstrual blood flow including endometrial shed tissue lasts 2–7 days [3, 4].

2 Endometrial Cyclic Changes

The endometrial cavity is a roughly triangular collapsed space, with the apex opening at the bottom into the endocervical canal's upper and internal ostium; the lower and external ostium of the endocervical canal opens into the vaginal cavity. The continuity of the endometrial cavity and the vagina makes possible the periodic shedding of the endometrial functional layer and of menstrual blood.

During the reproductive period of life, the endometrium undergoes cyclic changes that vary between 21 and 42 days, with the average cycle lasting 28 days. In this model, ovulation is presumed to occur on day 14. "Dating" of the endometrium is based on the histological description of the endometrial tissues, glands, stroma, and blood vessels every day of the cycle, starting after the menstrual shedding. The cyclic structural changes of the endometrial tissue occur under hormonal influences which are cyclic as well and dependent on a delicate balanced interplay of stimulation, withdrawal, and feedback between anterior pituitary, nonsteroid hormones, and gonadal (ovarian) steroid hormones, depending on the central nervous system, mostly hypothalamic factors. Ovarian follicles are selected each month by promoting the growth of one and atresia of the other graafian follicles. This is due to the secretion by the anterior pituitary lobe of follicular-stimulating hormone (FSH) during the stimulatory phase of the selected follicle. The granulosa cells in the follicles respond with the increase of their FSH receptors. The secretion of estradiol is related to granulosa aromatase synthesis depending on FSH arriving at the follicle and the ability of local estradiol to increase FSH receptors on follicle granulosa cells. FSH decline starts due to negative feedback at the preovulatory peak of increased estradiol and inhibin secretion. FSH-induced LH-receptor presence on the granulosa cells of the dominant follicle achieves LH stimulation at midcycle with subsequent progesterone synthesis on the cumulus and mural granulosa cells. LH initiates the process of ovulation and completion of meiosis, progressive luteinization of the follicle with granulosa cells shifting steroid synthesis to yield both estradiol and progesterone. Both enhance estradiol-positive feedback on GnRH pulse and anterior pituitary LH surge response. Eventually as the luteal phase progresses, progesterone-negative feedback acts to terminate the LH surge at both the pituitary and hypothalamic levels [5–8]. Gonadotropin releases at the maturation of the follicle are physiologically well coordinated based on feedback relationships, in the early follicle selection phase (FSH) and at ovulation (LH). The resulting "translation" by the endometrial tissue of hormonal cyclic stimulation and withdrawal is manifested at histologic examination by a prompt response consisting of a complex pattern of architectural and diversified cellular changes. "Dating" of these changes reflects the accuracy of adequate responses to hormones by the tissue destined to serve as a host to an implanting conceptus, thus securing the survival of the species.

The endometrial tissue lining the inner surface of the myometrium is composed of two layers: the basal layer and the functional layer. The basal layer lies on the myometrial tissue and is composed of basal glandular structures surrounded by stromal tissue containing blood vessels. It is poor in hormone receptors and does not display obvious structural changes during the menstrual cycle except for a partial shedding with the menstrual blood flow. During the reproductive life, the functional layer changes promptly exhibiting a wide variation of patterns involving glands, stroma, and blood vessels, with different aspects on every single day of the cycle, that can be assessed on endometrial biopsied tissue. During the preovulatory phase which lasts on average 14 days, but can be variable in its duration in otherwise normal cycles, the endometrium is proliferative under predominant estrogenic influence, and three consecutive patterns are described: early, mid-, and late proliferative endometrium. Specific histological patterns are expected to be seen on every single day of the postovulatory 14 days (for a summary of the histologic cyclic changes/"dating" of the endometrium, see Table 1).

The early proliferative phase starts with repair and regrowth of the endometrial tissues after menstrual shedding. Basal glands are proliferating from their bottom toward the surface, and the endometrial thickness increases up to tenfold during the preovulatory phase. The epithelial and stromal cells acquire estrogen receptors which are expressed during the proliferative and early secretory phase. The glands are tubular and straight lined by cuboidal to columnar epithelial cells in the early proliferative phase, become coiled in the mid-proliferative, and lined by columnar cells, and tortuous and pseudostratified in the late proliferative phase due to the

Table 1 Endometrial cyclic changes ("dating" of the endometrium)

Phase	Thickness	Glands	Epithelium	Nuclei	Stroma	Blood vessels	Mitoses
Early proliferative	1 mm	Straight tubular	Tall columnar	Centrally located mitoses nucleoli prominent	Abundant edema (day 8–10) scant cytoplasm (bare nuclei) mitoses	Thin straight inconspicuous	++
Mid-proliferative	8 mm	Coiled	Pseudostratified				
Late proliferative	10 mm	Tortuous					
Ovulation	12–15 mm	Tortuous coiled	Giant mitochondria	Plump, prominent chromatin	Edema	Thin, mildly coiled	+
Day 16	12–15 mm		Columnar, Subnuclear vacuoles	Middle third 50% "piano keys"	Spindle cells		+
Day 17	12–15 mm		Columnar, Supranuclear vacuoles	Middle third 90%			±
Day 18	12–15 mm	Intraglandular secretion	Frayed apical border	Basal			–
Day 19	12–15 mm		Cuboidal		Mild edema		–
Day 20	12–15 mm	Dilated, cystic					–
Day 21	12–15 mm	Dilated					–
Day 22	12–15 mm	Intraluminal secretion			Peak edema		–
Day 23	12–15 mm					Spiral arterioles	–
Day 24	12–15 mm				Perivascular decidua		–
Day 25	12–15 mm				Diffuse decidua		–
Day 26	12–15 mm	"Sawtooth" shape	Low cuboidal, exhausted				–
Day 27	8–10 mm		Apoptosis	Pyknotic	Leukocyte infiltrate breakdown	Fibrin thrombi	–
Day 28	2 mm	Disrupted secretory	Cell debris			Thrombosed	–
Early menstrual	1 mm		Apoptosis	Nuclear debris	Hemorrhage	Necrotic	–
Late menstrual	<1 mm	Necrotic					–

increase in size and numbers of the epithelial cells. Mitotic activity is also progressively increasing during the preovulatory phase. The nuclei of glandular epithelial cells are centrally located and display during early proliferation diffusely distributed chromatin. In mid- and late proliferative endometrium, the nuclei display coarse clumps of chromatin, and mitotic figures become frequent, located late in the apical region of the cells. Nucleoli are prominent, large, and complex. The apical border of the cell shows microvilli, and the cytoplasm contains abundant ribosomes reflecting the protein synthesis during the proliferative phase. The stroma is abundant, representing about half the volume of the endometrium, roughly equal to the volume of the glands. The stromal cells are spindle-shaped, with plump nuclei and scant cytoplasm; mitotic activity is present in the stroma along with that in the glands. There is stromal edema during the mid-proliferative phase, about on the eighth to tenth post menstrual day (Figs. 1 and 2). The blood vessels are rather inconspicuous, thin, and straight. Few hours after ovulation, the histologic appearance changes dramatically under the additional influence of progesterone secreted by the corpus luteum (Fig. 3). The endometrial tissue becomes more abundant, due to increase of stromal cells and edema. Histologically during the first postovulatory days, the endometrial glandular epithelium becomes secretory, first (day 16) showing subnuclear vacuoles (Figs. 4 and 5) which then, on the 17th day, become supranuclear. The epithelial cells on ultrastructure display giant mitochondria surrounded by loops of endoplasmic reticulum and glycogen accumulation in the sub- and supranuclear vacuoles (Fig. 6). The nuclei are pushed from their initial basal position to the middle third of the cell ("piano-key" image) and return on the 18th day to the basal position. During the proliferative phase, the endometrial surface is smooth; after ovulation, the secretory vacuoles are present in almost all (80–90%) cells lining all glands (Figs. 7 and 8). This is the histological evidence on endometrial biopsy that ovulation has indeed occurred and is an important finding in the work-up for infertility. By day 19–20, the vacuoles disappear from the cytoplasm being secreted at the luminal border into the glandular lumen. The apical border becomes frayed and the cell is cuboidal. No new mitoses are present in the glands during the secretory phase, except for those "leftover" during the first days from the proliferative phase. The stromal changes are most evident after day 20. Stromal edema is seen on day 21, reaching its peak on day 22, with stromal cells consisting of spindle-shaped nuclei and scant or visually absent cytoplasm (bare nuclei), while glands appear dilated, lined by a quiescent epithelium, containing abundant secretion in their lumen. On day 23 the vascular component of the endometrium, so far inconspicuous, becomes prominent with the appearance of spiral arterioles (Figs. 9 and 10). The coiled spiral arterioles increased in length and thickness and appear on histologic sections with multiple lumina, due to the coiling, with a markedly increased surface. This finding is important for the evaluation of the quality of the postovulatory endometrium. The coiled, increased surface of the endometrial arterioles offers more opportunity for a possible blastocystic trophoblast to tap into the maternal blood and achieve implantation. Endometrial biopsy evaluation for infertility assesses not only ovulation, evident as secretory glands, but its efficiency as a site of implantation, by the presence of well-formed spiral arterioles. On day 24 the stromal cells surrounding the spiral arterioles become decidualized: they become plump, and their central nuclei are surrounded by cytoplasm which increases in volume. This change extends to the stroma beyond the perivascular zones, involving the entire stroma by day 25. The decidual cells form a mosaiclike pattern with a compact endometrial surface. The glands after day 24 are dilated and contain inspissated secretion; on day 26 the glands have a sawtooth appearance, and their lining epithelium appears exhausted. On day 27 numerous leukocytes appear in the stroma, and the glandular epithelium exhibits fragmented nuclear debris due to the apoptosis of the tissue. On day 28 there is a marked infiltration of the stroma by leukocytes, and breakup by apoptosis of endometrial tissue starts. Dissolution of endometrial glands and stroma follows the withdrawal of both estrogens and progesterone as a result of negative feedback. On endometrial biopsy of early menstrual endometrium, there are disrupted glands with secretory features, though mostly exhausted, lined by cuboidal cells. Fibrin thrombi are seen in the blood vessels and the stroma appears broken down and hemorrhagic. During the following days of menstrual shedding and bleeding, the glands collapse, the stroma is condensed, and the nuclei become pyknotic. Endometrial biopsies taken at this point do not show sufficient evidence whether the cycle was ovulatory or not.

Dating of endometrium is the identification of the day of the cycle from the microscopic pattern of endometrial biopsies. An accurate evaluation is possible due to the specific features that are characteristic for each postovulatory day and for most proliferative days. Diagnosing the presence and quality of ovulation from its endometrial tissue response is an important test for the adequacy of this tissue as a potential host for an implanting conceptus. Iatrogenic hormone therapy, mostly steroid sex hormone therapy, has an important influence on the endometrial micro-

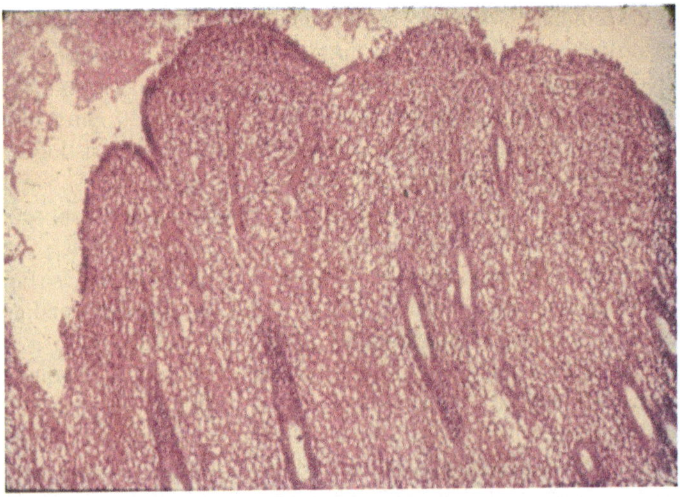

Fig. 1 Mid-proliferative endometrium: glands are straight, stroma edematous. H&E ×40

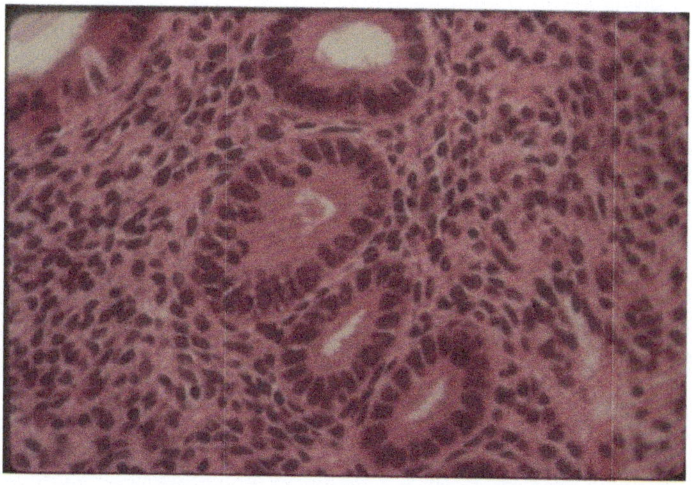

Fig. 2 Mid-proliferative endometrium: tubular glands. Mitotic activity in the glands H&E x 100

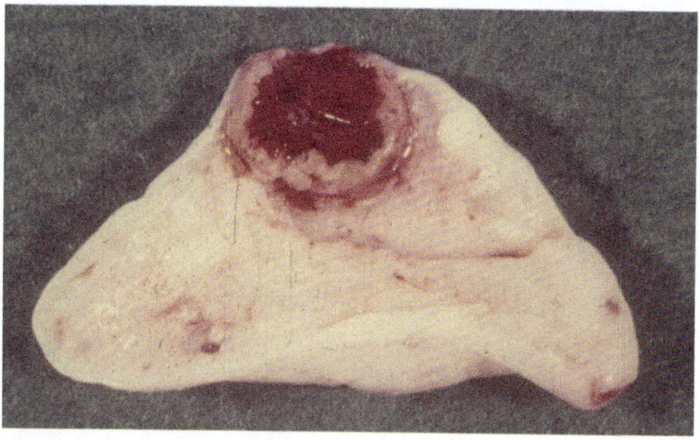

Fig. 3 Ovulating ovary with hemorrhagic corpus luteum

structure modifying the histologic patterns and often creating confusion when compared to the natural cyclic changes.

3 Uterus at Menopause

Menopause is characterized by the progressive diminution and eventual cessation of ovarian secretion of estrogen, due to failure to respond to gonadotropic hormones. Within a year after the final menstrual period, ovarian follicle exhaustion is complete. FSH and LH continue to rise with tripling of LH by 3 years postmenopause.

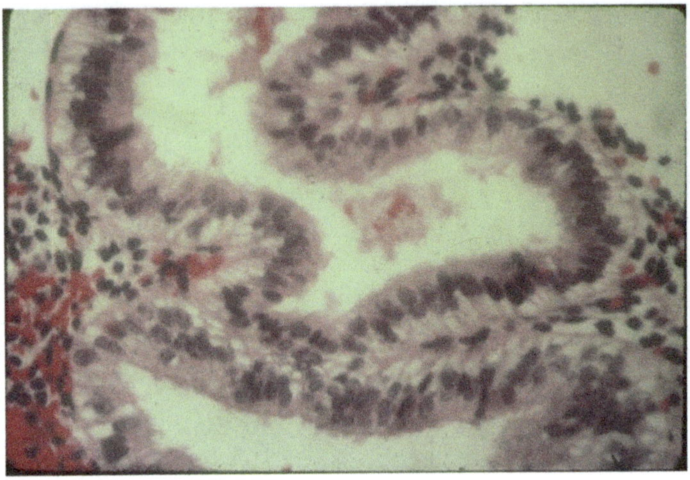

Fig. 4 Postovulatory endometrium: day 16–17 subnuclear vacuoles. H&E ×40

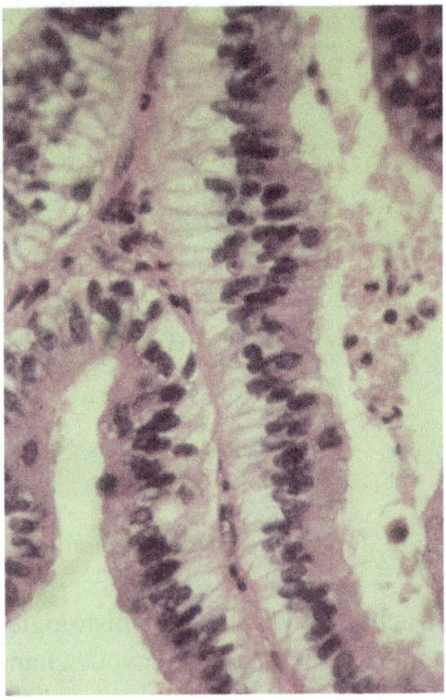

Fig. 5 Postovulatory endometrium, day 16–17. Subnuclear vacuoles, nuclei in middle third of cell, "piano-key" pattern H&E x100

Hypergonadotropism persists, although diminished [9]. In the absence of estrogen stimulation, the endometrium becomes thin, inactive (non-proliferative and nonsecretory), and gradually atrophic. The myometrium including possible leiomyomas is shrinking as well. The endometrium is thin, less than 1 mm. On endometrial biopsies the glands appear straight, tubular, and lined by cuboidal epithelium with centrally located round nuclei. No pseudostratification is present. Commonly seen are cystically dilated glands lined by flattened epithelium [10]. On ultrastructure the

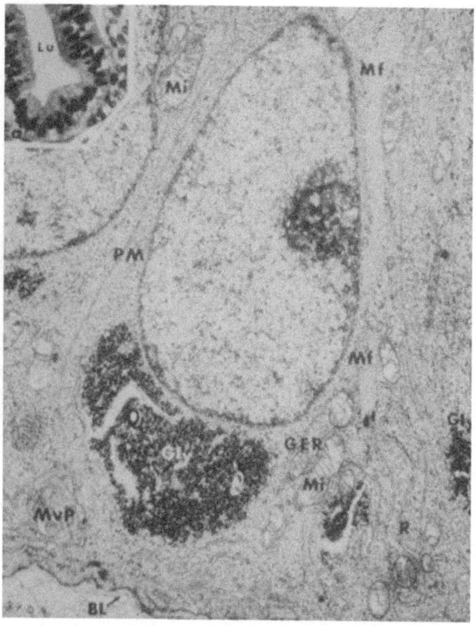

Fig. 6 Transmission electron microscopic image of postovulatory endometrium: subnuclear glycogen aggregates, prominent nucleolus, large mitochondria surrounded by endoplasmic reticulum, free cytoplasmic ribosomes

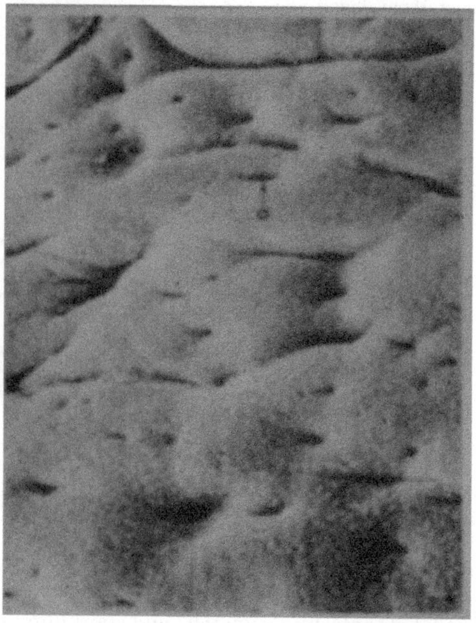

Fig. 7 Scanning electron microscopy: proliferative endometrium. Note smooth surface and glandular openings

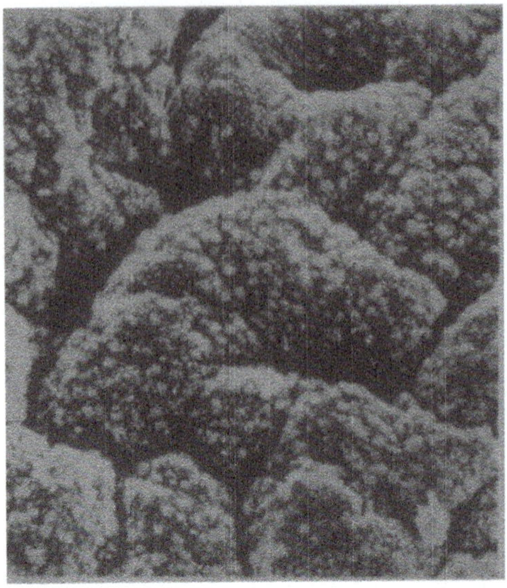

Fig. 8 Scanning electron microscopy: secretory endometrium, deeply folded surface covered by secretory granules

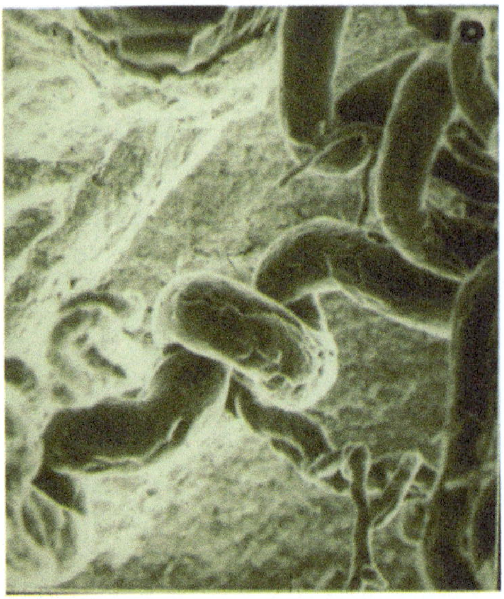

Fig. 9 Scanning electron microscopy: spiral arterioles on day 23

cytoplasmic organelles are poorly developed and randomly distributed, with occasional cytoplasmic vacuoles, and short blunt microvilli are noted on the apical border of the cells [11]. The stroma is dense with a network of precollagen fibers surrounding spindle-shaped cells, with an occasional lymphoid cell infiltrate. Perimenopausal irregular vaginal bleeding is common, and endometrial biopsies may show glandular crowding due to stromal breakdown. The crowding and back-

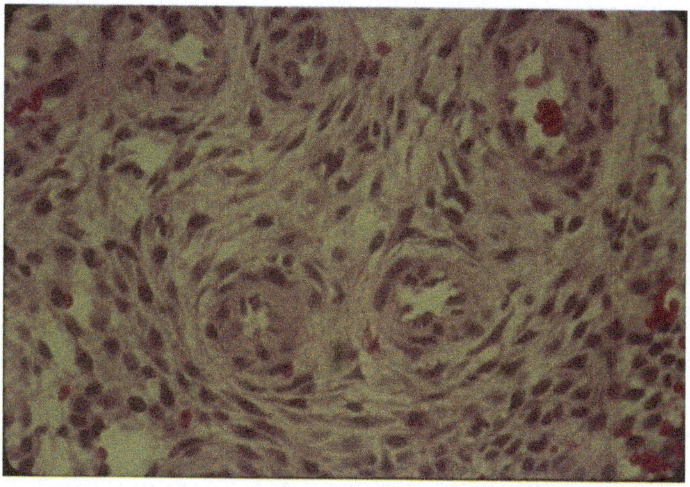

Fig. 10 Spiral arteriole surrounded by decidualized stromal cells, day 24, H&E x 100

to-back glandular pattern may arise suspicions of hyperplasia and neoplasia. Careful examination of the epithelial cells to identify nuclear atypia (different from "smudged" nuclei), special stains for p53, K67, and estrogen/progesterone receptors are helpful for the diagnosis and further management of the patient, including hormone therapy for menopause. Extragonadal estrogen in postmenopausal women is derived from androgen conversion to estrogen. Available estrogen varies with the substrate; as the amount of fat and the aromatase capacity of fat tissue increase, circulating levels of total and free estrone and estradiol increase [12–15]. With obesity sex hormone-binding globulin levels decrease providing greater androgen substrate availability and higher concentration of free biologically active estrogens [16–19].

Endometrial biopsies are frequently performed on peri- and postmenopausal women, in order to establish the nature of often occurring irregular vaginal bleeding, to rule out possible malignancy or precursor of malignant changes, and to establish a baseline before hormone replacement therapy (HRT) is recommended. The interpretation of the histologic findings may be difficult as hormonal influences are often unpredictable during the process of ovarian gradual failure, and locally, the hormone receptors may be irregularly distributed or absent. Given the wide variety of histopathologic and immunopathologic patterns, the management of the patient, hormone therapy including HRT, has to be individualized and coordinated with the general state of health and metabolism (especially obesity and diabetes) and correlated with the baseline endometrial biopsy.

References

1. Bazer FW, Roberts RM, Thatcher WW. Actions of hormones on the uterus and effect of conceptus development. J Anim Sci. 1979;49(Suppl 2):35–45.
2. O'Brien Y, Wingfield M, O'Shea LC. Anti-Müllerian hormone and progesterone levels in human follicular fluid are predictors of embryonic development. Reprod Biol Endocrinol. 2019;17(1):47. https://doi.org/10.1186/s12958-019-0492-9.
3. Brosens I, Benagiano G. The endometrium from the neonate to the adolescent. J Matern Fetal Neonatal Med. 2016;29(8):1195–9.
4. Fritz MA, Speroff L. The endocrinology of the menstrual cycle: the interaction of folliculogenesis and neuroendocrine mechanisms. Fertil Steril. 1982;38(5):509–29. Review.
5. Mais V, Kazer RR, Cetel NS, Rivier J, Vale W, Yen SS. The dependency of folliculogenesis and corpus luteum function on pulsatile gonadotropin secretion in cycling women using a gonadotropin-releasing hormone antagonist as a probe. J Clin Endocrinol Metab. 1986;62(6):1250–5.
6. Kase NG. The normal human ovary. In: Altchek A, editor. Diagnosis and management of ovarian disorders. 3rd ed. Cambridge University Press; 2013.
7. Hansen KR, Knowlton NS, Thyer AC, Charleston JS, Soules MR, Klein NA. A new model of reproductive aging: the decline in ovarian non-growing follicle number from birth to menopause. Hum Reprod. 2008;23(3):699–708.
8. Gougeon A, Ecochard R, Thalabard JC. Age-related changes of the population of human ovarian follicles: increase in the disappearance rate of non-growing and early-growing follicles in aging women. Biol Reprod. 1994;50(3):653–63.
9. Kase NG. Menopause. In: Altchek A, editor. Diagnosis and management of ovarian disorders. 3rd ed. Cambridge University Press; 2013.
10. Feldman S, Shapter A, Welch WR, Berkowitz RS. Two-year follow-up of 263 patients with post/perimenopausal vaginal bleeding and negative initial biopsy. Gynecol Oncol. 1994;55(1):56–9.
11. Deligdisch L, Yedwab G, Persitz A, David MP. Ultrastructural features in normal and hyperplastic postmenopausal endometrium. Acta Obstet Gynecol Scand. 1978;57(5):439–52.
12. Harlow SD, Gass M, Hall JE, Lobo R, Maki P, Rebar RW, Sherman S, Sluss PM, de Villiers TJ, STRAW + 10 Collaborative Group. Executive summary of the Stages of Reproductive Aging Workshop + 10: addressing the unfinished agenda of staging reproductive aging. Fertil Steril. 2012;97(4):843–51.
13. McKinlay SM, Bifano NL, McKinlay JB. The normal menopause transition. Maturitas. 1992;14(2):103–15.
14. Gosden RG, Faddy MJ. Ovarian aging, follicular depletion, and steroidogenesis. Exp Gerontol. 1994;29(3–4):265–74. Review.
15. Randolph JF Jr, Zheng H, Sowers MR, Crandall C, Crawford S, Gold EB, Vuga M. Change in follicle-stimulating hormone and estradiol across the menopausal transition: effect of age at the final menstrual period. J Clin Endocrinol Metab. 2011;96(3):746–54.
16. Burger HG, Dudley EC, Cui J, Dennerstein L, Hopper JL. A prospective longitudinal study of serum testosterone, dehydroepiandrosterone sulfate, and sex hormone-binding globulin levels through the menopause transition. J Clin Endocrinol Metab. 2000;85(8):2832–8.
17. Janssen I, Powell LH, Crawford S, Lasley B, Sutton-Tyrrell K. Menopause and the metabolic syndrome: the study of Women's Health Across the Nation. Arch Intern Med. 2008;168(14):1568–75.
18. Carr MC. The emergence of the metabolic syndrome with menopause. J Clin Endocrinol Metab. 2003;88(6):2404–11. Review.
19. Flegal KM. Prevalence of obesity and trends in the distribution of body mass index among US adults, 1999–2010. JAMA. 2012;307(5):491–7.

Hormonal Effects in Reproductive Technology with Focus on Diminished Ovarian Reserve

David Barad

1 Introduction

We often take our biological functions for granted. When a natural function ceases to occur normally, we feel cheated, betrayed by our own bodies. This is never truer than when a couple finds themselves dealing with the problem of infertility.

Infertility has been defined as the failure to achieve an ongoing pregnancy within the course of 1 year of trying to conceive. But in fact, for couples who have decided to build a family, each month without an established pregnancy can feel like a little death. Since reproduction is commonly dependent on sexual intercourse between a man and woman, in the past, it was relegated to a very private sphere of discussion. For decades couples suffered privately with this problem, too embarrassed to discuss it with their families or even with their physicians.

A deeper understanding of reproductive processes has evolved in our lifetime to encompass greater control of reproduction, both in contraception and in family building, and has gradually brought this conversation into the open and provided new tools to help couples faced with these problems.

Reproductive problems that, in the past, were often surgically treated can now be approached with less intervention. Men and women who, in the past, would be left childless can now find hope to build their families. This chapter will describe some of the tools we now use to help couples achieve their family goals, especially those dealing with diminished ovarian reserve, and will look at how we expect these opportunities to grow in the future.

D. Barad (✉)
Mt Sinai West, New York, NY, USA

Center for Human Reproduction (CHR), New York, NY, USA
e-mail: dbarad@thechr.com

L. Deligdisch-Schor, A. Mareş Miceli (eds.), *Hormonal Pathology of the Uterus*, Advances in Experimental Medicine and Biology 1242,
https://doi.org/10.1007/978-3-030-38474-6_2

2 Causes of Infertility

In simplest terms there are three major components in evaluating the infertile couple: (1) evaluation of normal sperm production and function, (2) evaluation of normal ovarian production of oocytes, and (3) evaluation of anatomical factors that might prevent the joining of these gametes.

2.1 *Male Factor*

Semen analysis should be one of the first evaluations undertaken. Male factor infertility is present in half of all infertile couples [1]. Evaluation by means of a semen analysis is inexpensive and noninvasive. Today, most cases of male factor infertility can be addressed using assisted reproductive technologies; however, male factor will not be a major focus of this chapter.

2.2 *Tubal Factor*

Today, instead of undergoing tubal surgery, it is more likely for a patient to choose in-vitro fertilization to achieve pregnancy. Today's reproductive surgeons are not likely to experience many tubal ligation reversals or even lysis of adhesions as part of their training. Surgical correction of tubal infertility has become a thing of the past as the generation of surgeons trained in those procedures is aging out of practice and IVF techniques and laboratories continue to improve. Instead, the surgeons in training are more likely to find themselves performing a salpingectomy or proximal tubal ligation in order to improve pregnancy rates with IVF [2, 3]. While such surgery can improve the odds of a successful IVF cycle, benefit of this improvement must be weighed against the risks of surgery. Women undergoing IVF after salpingectomy may not respond as well to ovulation induction [4], though this change in response may have little clinical importance for a woman beginning with normal ovarian reserve, it may well have clinical importance for those who already have evidence of diminished ovarian reserve. In our practice, where most of our patients have diminished functional ovarian reserve, we rarely recommend tubal surgery before undergoing IVF.

2.3 *Ovarian Reserve*

A thorough understanding of ovarian physiology is needed to understand and treat problems of ovarian reserve. Women are born with all the oocytes they will ever have. Primordial follicles form during the first 5 months of fetal development. At birth a woman may have up to four million primordial follicles; however, by puberty these numbers will have diminished to only 200,000–400,000. This cohort is further depleted each month, and, in a woman's late 30s, when the total cohort has fallen below 25,000, loss of follicles continues to fall even more rapidly eventually reaching menopausal levels when there are fewer than 1000 follicles at around age 51 [5].

Throughout life primordial follicles (the oocyte surrounded by a thin layer of follicular epithelial cells) will represent most follicles in the ovary. As follicles transition from primordial to primary, secondary, tertiary, and ultimately graafian follicle stages, most will be lost. Over a women's reproductive lifetime only 400–600 of these follicles will ever achieve ovulation. Thus, for every follicle that achieves ovulation, thousands will have degenerated into atresia. The process of selection as follicles transition toward maturity can take several months and may be thought of in three basic stages: gonadotropin-independent pre-antral follicles, gonadotropin-dependent antral follicles, and growing graafian follicles. Each of these stages has specific characteristics and opportunities for clinical manipulation, although in general only the last (graafian follicle) stage has been subject to treatment in the past.

The clinical index of the ability of the ovary to produce oocytes is known as functional ovarian reserve (FOR) which is generally dependent on the antral follicle pool. Age is the primary marker of ovarian reserve; however, in any given age group, there may be a wide range of FOR that can be estimated by other predictors in addition to age [6]. Some predictors of FOR, other than a woman's age, are antral follicle count (AFC), anti-Mullerian hormone (AMH), and cycle basal follicle-stimulating hormone (b-FSH) level.

2.3.1 Antral Follicle Count (AFC)

Antral follicles are those follicles variously defined as being between 4 and 10 mm in diameter. The antral follicle is characterized by having a fluid-filled antrum. Antral follicles are gonadotropin dependent, and, under influence of LH, antral thecal cells secrete androgens that, together with circulating androgen from the adrenal cortex, can then, under influence of FSH, be aromatized to estrogen by the neighboring granulosa cells.

Modern sonography allows the recognition of the small developing antral follicles in the ovary. Antral follicle count (AFC) may be used as an index of a woman's ovarian reserve. A normal AFC is between 4 and 24 follicles between 2 and 10 mm in diameter [7]. Both AFC and ovarian volume decrease with age; however, AFC has been shown to be a better predictor of poor ovarian response than ovarian volume [8]. An AFC of less than four was associated with an almost nine times lower chance of achieving a pregnancy with IVF [9]. Having a higher AFC is associated with an increased risk of ovarian hyperstimulation syndrome [10]; this risk increases continuously with increased AFC, though there is no established consistent cutoff for risk of hyperstimulation.

2.3.2 Basal Follicle-Stimulating Hormone (b-FSH)

For more than 30 years, basal follicle-stimulating hormone has been used to estimate ovarian reserve and a woman's potential to achieve pregnancy [11–13]. Basal FSH (b-FSH) is an indirect measure of ovarian reserve since it is measuring the hypothalamic-pituitary response to feedback from developing ovarian antral follicles which secrete activins, inhibins, and follistatins in addition sex steroids [14]. The testing is done on day 2 or 3 of the menstrual cycle since the ovarian sex steroids from developing follicles are at their lowest level at that time. Because of this the b-FSH level reflects the feedback of the other peptides more than that of the sex steroids. When the b-FSH testing is done, it is necessary to also measure estradiol simultaneously to confirm that estradiol is at a basal level, less than 60 pg/mL. As women age there are fewer antral follicles producing substances to inhibit FSH, and as a result, basal FSH will steadily rise. In general women with levels of b-FSH less than 10–12 mIU/mL are considered to have "normal" ovarian reserve, and those with higher levels are considered to be potential "poor responders" [13, 15]. The highest b-FSH a woman has had is a better predictor than a current b-FSH of her response in any treatment cycle [16, 17], and waiting for a cycle with more favorable lower b-FSH does not improve IVF outcomes.

The concept of age-specific testing considers that there is a specific normal range for b-FSH for each age group (Fig. 1). Age-specific b-FSH levels can be a useful guide in measuring a woman's ovarian reserve at any age [18–20]. Age-specific testing allows the adjustment of planned ovulation induction protocols appropriate for

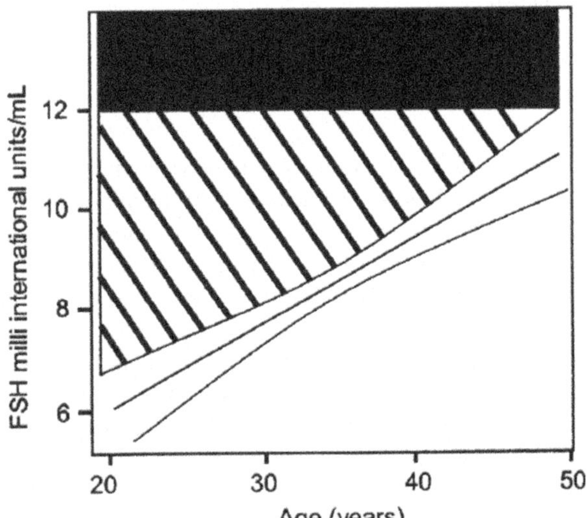

Fig. 1 Cycle day-3 baseline follicle-stimulating hormone mean 95% confidence interval by age. Shaded area superimposed on figure to illustrate patients identified with premature ovarian aging (diagonal lines) or diminished ovarian reserve (black). (From Barad. Age-Specific Ovarian Function Testing. Obstet Gynecol 2007)

a woman's specific ovarian reserve [21]. Too often an b-FSH greater than 12 is used to recommend the use of donor eggs rather than a women's own [22]. In our practice we have found that women with b-FSH greater than 20 mIU/mL can still achieve live birth rates of up to 6% per initiated IVF cycle [23]. While such rates are still far lower than those that could be anticipated using eggs of a younger donor, we believe that couples should have a right to choose what they feel is the best option for them.

2.3.3 Anti-Mullerian Hormone (AMH)

Anti-Mullerian hormone (AMH) is a glycoprotein hormone in the transforming growth factor family and is a product of pre-antral and small antral follicles. Since AMH is produced by each pre-antral and small antral follicle, the serum AMH levels can be used as an index of the functional ovarian reserve, not reflecting the entire ovarian cohort of follicles but only those in the antral follicle stage [24–27]. These follicles are, indeed, those that are about to enter competition for graafian follicle dominance.

As follicles approach the antral stage, they gain the ability to produce anti-Mullerian hormone (AMH). AMH plays an important role in regulating follicular development. High levels of AMH will inhibit the transition of early follicle stages to the antral stage and will inhibit FSH stimulation of antral follicle transition to graafian follicles [28]. Once follicles transition to the graafian follicle stage, they no longer have the capacity to produce AMH. Any factor that will influence the antral follicle cohort will be reflected in changes in AMH serum levels. Both recent pregnancy and use of strong hormonal contraception can lower AMH levels [29, 30]. Serum levels of AMH decrease as a woman ages, and the number of antral follicles and functional ovarian reserve is decreased. Consequently age-specific levels of AMH can be used to judge a woman's current state of FOR relative to her peers [25, 31, 32].

3 Ovulation Induction

More than 40 years ago, the first successful IVF cycle was conducted without ovulation induction [33]. It soon became clear that success in IVF could be improved by recruiting as many oocytes as possible [34]. Thereafter, therapeutic strategies originally used to treat an ovulatory women were transitioned to the treatment of ovulatory women. In nature the human ovulatory cycle allows the promotion of only one, or rarely two, graafian follicle to reach maturity and ovulate. Exogenous administration of gonadotropins to an ovulatory woman was used to raise the level of follicle-stimulating hormone high enough that the full cohort of gonadotropin-dependent follicles was allowed to grow and mature leading to the production of multiple oocytes [35]. This type of controlled ovarian stimulation (COS) created a greater chance of conception and a parallel consequent increase in the risk of multiple pregnancy if conception was allowed in vivo.

It soon became clear that the cumulative likelihood of live birth with IVF increases with the number of oocytes retrieved [36–38]. Increased rates of live birth were even more apparent when taking cumulative pregnancy rate (fresh plus subsequent transfer of cryopreserved embryos) into account [37, 39].

When using COS for IVF, dosing of FSH generally ranges from 150 to 450 IU with the dose often adjusted according to estimated ovarian reserve based on age, antral follicle count (AFC), anti-Mullerian hormone (AMH), and day-3 FSH. The intent of such individualized COS is to produce an effective number of mature oocytes with minimal risk of hyperstimulation or other complications. Among women with good ovarian reserve, increased gonadotropin dosage will lead to increased recovery of oocytes [40] and a subsequent improved live birth rate, as noted above.

However, past experience has shown that for woman with evidence of decreased ovarian reserve, the use of increased gonadotropin doses alone to achieve greater oocyte recovery is often futile [41, 42]. One study of indicators of ovarian reserve found that there is great individual variation in response to COS that appears to be independent of these predictors [43]. Another found that while women with diminished FOR had greater risk of cancelation of their IVF cycles, those who reached transfer had only a small, though significant, decreased adjusted relative risk of live birth [44]. A meta-analysis found that IVF live birth rates with individualized COS did not differ significantly from live birth rates when 150 units of FSH was administered no matter what the assessed ovarian reserve [45]. Thus, the use of individualized COS remains controversial. In our practice we believe that response to ovulation induction is most dependent on the functional ovarian reserve (FOR) which is in turn dependent on maintenance of the antral follicle pool.

4 Maintenance of the Antral Follicle Pool

A good antral follicle pool is essential for providing best chance of reproductive success [46–48]. Antral follicles are the resource from which graafian follicles will develop. Past approaches to ovulation induction focused on promotion of antral follicles into graafian follicle growth by provision of excess gonadotropin either by exogenous injection of gonadotropins or by inducing production of endogenous gonadotropin by inhibiting normal feedback to the pituitary of hypothalamus [49].

Women lose ovarian reserve as they age through the depletion of their remaining follicles and consequent diminished replenishment of the antral follicle pool. With fewer antral follicles, fewer graafian follicles can develop. As the population of developing follicles is diminished, so too is the endocrine milieu of the ovary. This leads to a variety of other consequences for the reproductive system in general including progressive symptoms of sex hormone deprivation such as vaginal dryness, loss of libido, hot flashes, and sleep disturbance.

Over the past decade, our group has explored various ways of helping women to get the most function out of their remaining follicle pool. The underlying philosophy of this approach is to foster the preservation and growth of pre-antral and antral follicles to provide maintenance of the antral follicle pool.

4.1 Factors Promoting Growth of Pre-antral and Antral Follicles

4.1.1 Androgens

In women circulating androgens are derived from both the adrenal glands and the ovaries [50]. The major adrenal androgens are dehydroepiandrosterone (DHEA) and its sulfate DHEAS which are produced in the zona reticularis of the human adrenal cortex [51]. With age the number of cells in the zona reticularis is known to decrease leading to decreased production of DHEA and DHEAS [51–53]. Androgens are precursors required for normal ovarian steroidogenesis [54, 55]. Thus, with loss of adrenal androgen production, there is a consequent loss of ovarian function.

Androgens are important growth factors for early follicle development. Support for the concept that androgens are necessary for normal early follicular development comes from experiments using androgen receptor knockout mouse models [56, 57]. In these experiments granulosa cell-specific androgen receptor knockout (ARKO) mice were used to examine the role of androgens in normal follicular development. GC-specific ARKO mice were more likely than wild type to have ovarian failure and longer estrous cycles. In addition, ovaries from the GC-specific ARKO mice had a greater proportion of pre-antral and atretic follicles with evidence of fewer antral follicles or corpora lutea [57]. In later studies androgens were found to decrease follicular atresia by suppression of proapoptotic protein expression and enhancement of FSH receptor expression, independent of transcription [58]. Similar non-genomic modulation of androgen action has been reported in other species [59].

In the setting of excess androgens, more follicles can develop to the antral follicle stage. One consequence of this androgen excess is the typical picture of polycystic ovary syndrome in which excess androgens lead to an excess number of antral follicles and excessively high AMH. The high AMH levels interfere with the action of follicle-stimulating hormone and may contribute to anovulation.

Recognition of this interaction of androgens and antral follicle growth has led to the use of androgens to promote greater numbers of follicles to the antral follicle stage in women who have diminished ovarian reserve. This approach presumes that there are still pre-antral follicles that could be promoted.

We first became aware of this phenomenon while treating a patient who was almost 43 years old and was undergoing back-to-back oocyte banking cycles. In her first few cycles, she produced only one or two oocytes, but then, after a few more cycles, her oocyte production increased markedly ultimately producing 17 oocytes in her eighth consecutive treatment cycle [60]. When we observed the remarkable increase in production of oocytes, we asked what she might be doing that was promoting this response. She told us that she had begun using dehydroepiandrosterone (DHEA) after her early cycles had failed to produce many oocytes. She became aware of the potential for DHEA to augment ovarian response to ovulation induction by reading an earlier series of case reports on the internet [61].

Following this experience, we began offering DHEA to other patients with evidence of diminished ovarian reserve and found that in a remarkable number of cases we were able to make a significant difference in response and in pregnancy rates [62, 63]. Recent meta-analyses have concluded that in women reported to be poor responders, pre-treatment with DHEA or testosterone may be associated with improved IVF live birth rates [64, 65].

There are a few important caveats in using DHEA among women with poor ovarian reserve. It is important not to heavily suppress gonadotropins in the preparatory phase of treatment. Effectiveness of androgen treatment appears to be partly dependent on the interaction of androgens and the endogenous gonadotropins. This may be a possible explanation why some trials of DHEA in which long agonist IVF protocol was used have been unable to show a significant benefit of DHEA treatment [66].

We do not use oral contraceptives to schedule IVF cycles. The use of oral contraceptives to help schedule cycles may lead to a 20% reduction in live birth rate [67]. The use of oral contraceptives has been associated with reduction in the antral follicle pool [68] and can reduce IVF oocyte yields [29].

In our practice the current preferred approach is for patients with diminished ovarian reserve to use micronized DHEA 25 mg three times a day for up to 2 months prior to initiation of ovulation induction. We prefer our patients to use divided doses because DHEA is rapidly absorbed and rapidly cleared and we would like to provide a steady blood level. We test for serum androgens and ovarian reserve parameters before starting DHEA and at baseline for each menstrual cycle. In general, in the presence of SHBG around 50–60 nmol/L, our target for total testosterone is between 28 and 56 ng/dL (1.0–2.0 nmol/L). We found that most of our patients with diminished ovarian reserve had baseline testosterone of less than 20 ng/dL and that only those who were able to raise testosterone to approach a minimal level of 30 ng/dL had favorable results to treatment [69].

4.1.2 Growth Hormone

Growth hormone is a hormone secreted by the somatotroph cells of the anterior pituitary peptide hormone important for cell growth, normal development, and metabolism. Growth hormone acts on the liver to produce IGF-1, which is responsible for growth hormone's metabolic effects. IGF-1 receptors are present both in human oocytes and cumulus granulosa cells [70–72]. IGF-1 has been shown to have a role in murine granulosa cell differentiation [73], follicle recruitment [74], oocyte maturation and FSH receptor development [75], and inhibition of apoptosis [76]. IGF-1 increases the estradiol secretory response of granulosa cells to follicle-stimulating hormone [77]. In women undergoing IVF, the level of follicular fluid IGF-1 was found to be proportional to the number of oocytes retrieved and inversely proportional to the amount of gonadotropin needed for successful ovulation induction [78]. Co-treatment with growth hormone was found to be associated with increased density of FSH receptors, LH receptors, bone morphogenetic hormone receptors, and growth hormone receptors of granulosa cells of older women with a history of poor ovarian reserve [79].

Growth hormone supplementation is potentially useful in ovulation induction. Over the last decades as recombinant growth hormone has become commercially available, there have been many studies looking at the effects of growth hormone on ovulation induction [80–86]. Almost all these studies administered growth hormone along with routine fertility medication during the ovulation induction cycle. Most studies used GH doses between 4 and 12 units per day. A few studies started GH on day 21 of the previous cycle. Evidence for meta-analysis has suggested that growth hormone has the greatest benefit when used to treat women classed as poor responders, those with a history of fewer than four oocytes retrieved in a previous cycle.

Recent randomized trials in poor responders have confirmed a growth hormone benefit in increased collected oocytes; however, growth hormone had no effect on the primary outcome of live birth [87, 88].

A recent Cochrane review found that while GH did not improve results in routine IVF cycles there is "some evidence of increased pregnancy and birth rates in women who are considered 'poor responders' to in vitro fertilization."

Growth hormone is reported to modulate the action of FSH on follicles by upregulating local synthesis of IGF-1. Interestingly a similar effect was noted by Casson [61, 89] in early experiments using DHEA with treated patients having increased IGF-1. Much of the focus on gonadotropin/IGF-1 interaction has revolved around the effects on granulosa cell cultures to increase aromatase activity, estradiol production, progesterone production, and LH receptor formation. However, IGF-1 also has a proposed role in stimulating early follicle development and oocyte maturation [90, 91].

Synthetic human growth hormone was developed in 1985 and approved by the FDA for specific uses in children and adults. Synthetic growth hormone use as a supplement for ovulation induction has not been FDA approved.

We believe the greatest potential for GH would be during preparation for an ovulation induction cycle. Theoretically administration of GH during the 6 weeks before starting a cycle will influence developing antral follicles to present a better cohort of follicles when ovulation induction is begun.

4.1.3 Platelet-Rich Plasma

As women age oocytes are gradually depleted with a consequent progressive loss of ovarian function and fertility. When a woman's follicle cohort falls below a critical level, she enters a transitional time of diminished ovarian reserve known as ovarian insufficiency. For most women this phase begins in the mid to late 30s and may last over 10–15 years before the onset of actual menopause. During this transition fertility is continuously reduced as is the production of ovarian sex steroids leading to increased symptoms of estrogen deficiency. These changes naturally occur at a time in their lives when contemporary women may only just be beginning to think about having a family.

Various strategies have been applied to help women restore ovarian function or to maximize the utility of what function may remain. Most past approaches to treatment of ovarian insufficiency have focused on maximizing induction of the cohort of antral follicles which constitute a women's functional ovarian reserve. These are the follicles which have survived the several months of development from primordial follicle to the antral follicle stage and most likely represent only a fraction of that original cohort.

Recently the use of platelet-rich plasma (PRP) has been proposed as an additional strategy for improving ovarian function [89]. PRP has been used in other medical fields to regenerate skin [90] and cartilage [91]. The rational for the use of PRP in these settings is that it contains growth factors which stimulate cellular anabolism, inflammatory modulators that create an anti-inflammatory effect, and fibrinogen which acts as a scaffold for regenerating tissue [92–94].

One current hypothesis regarding the possible effect of PRP in the ovary is that the growth factors released by activated PRP may induce the transformation of germline stem cells (GSCs) into primordial follicles, thus replenishing a diminished follicle pool [95]. Evidence in support of this hypothesis is limited [89, 96–98]. A few case reports of pregnancies occurring in women said to have premature ovarian failure have recently been reported [89, 99].

Women with POI may still have occasional irregular periods and may even occasionally achieve a pregnancy. In our practice we are presently recruiting women with POI into a clinical trial (NCT03542708) in which one randomly selected ovary is treated with PRP and the other ovary remains as a control. The endpoint of this study is to see if there is a differential response in follicle development between the treated and untreated ovary.

4.1.4 Estrogen Priming

We use estrogen priming for 7–10 days before beginning ovulation induction. Once ovulation induction is begun, we switch the estrogen prime to ethinylestradiol, which does not interfere with assay reading of estradiol coming from the patient's ovaries.

5 Optimizing Oocyte Production

5.1 *Individualized Egg Retrieval*

Over the past 2 years, we rarely used any cycle control at all. Instead we time our retrievals earlier than spontaneous ovulation would be expected to occur in the protocol we have called highly individualized egg retrieval [103].

As women age, oocyte quantity [5] and quality [104] are significantly diminished. Among older women undergoing ovulation induction for in vitro fertilization, a large percentage of oocytes retrieved are atretic [105]. The bidirectional communication in the cumulus granulosa cells and the oocyte is critical for the oocytes growth and differentiation [106–108]. With aging, the number of cumulus granulosa cells per oocyte [109] and the competence of those cells to maintain oocyte health become compromised [110].

We found that granulosa cell molecular function was diminished among older women. FSH receptor (FSHR), aromatase (CYP19A1), and 17b-hydroxysteroid dehydrogenase (HSD17B) expression were downregulated, while LH receptor (LHCGR), P450scc (CYP11A1), and progesterone receptor (PGR) were upregulated in granulosa cells collected from follicular fluid of women undergoing in vitro fertilization cycles. Together these findings revealed age-related changes consistent with premature luteinization [105] (Fig. 2).

We reasoned that loss of cumulus granulosa cell support could be a direct cause of the increasing incidence of oocyte atresia observed among our older patients. Based on this observation, we began timing retrieval at earlier stages of follicular development among older women [105]. This change in timing of oocyte retrieval resulted in a lower percentage of atretic eggs and a significantly improved pregnancy rate [103] (Table 1).

5.2 *In Vitro Maturation of Immature Oocytes (IVM)*

One consequence of moving the timing of the oocyte retrieval to earlier stages of follicular development is that a greater percentage of oocytes are MI or GV. We chose to retrieve immature oocytes rather than atretic oocytes that had no possibility of salvage. As expected, many of the MI oocytes progressed to MII once the cumulus granulosa cells were stripped away. Although these oocytes achieve nuclear maturity, they may not have achieved cytoplasmic maturity, and thus embryos produced from these in vitro oocytes do not have the same potential to achieve pregnancy as those oocytes that were already MII at collection. Clearly, this is an area that will need more exploration.

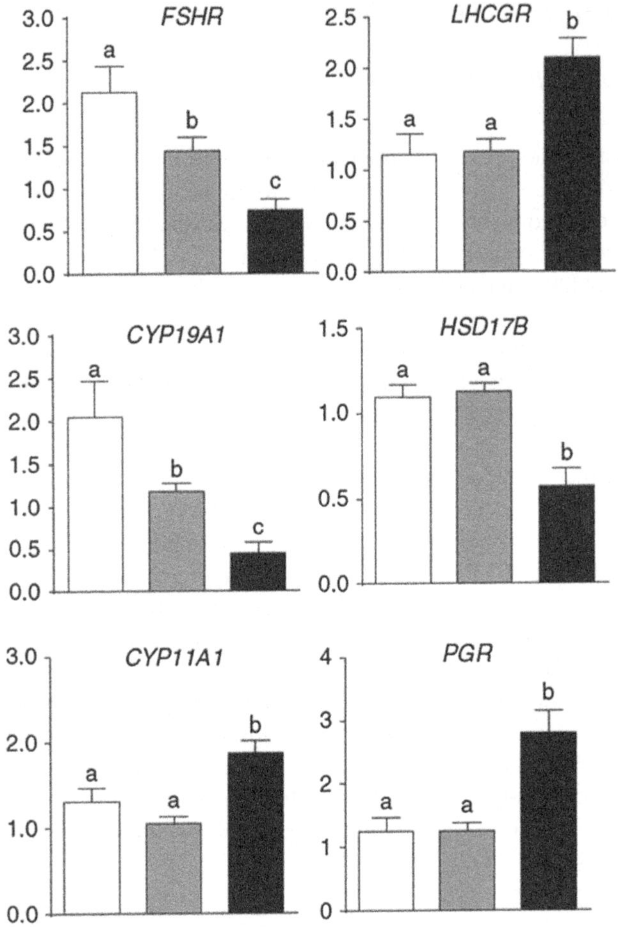

Fig. 2 mRNA expression of genes from granulosa cells collected from follicular fluid of women undergoing in vitro fertilization cycles determined by real-time PCR. Values with same letters or without letters above the columns within each unit figure were not different significantly (PO0.05). White columns: group 1 (oocyte donors), $n = 7$; gray columns: group 2 (middle-aged infertile patients), $n = 10$; black columns: group 3 (older infertile patients), $n = 10$. (*FSH receptor (FSHR), aromatase (CYP19A1), 17b-hydroxysteroid dehydrogenase (HSD17B) LH receptor (LHCGR), P450scc (CYP11A1), and progesterone receptor (PGR)*). (Adapted from Wu, Barad et al. J Endocrinol. 2015 Sep;226(3):167–80)

5.3 *Rebound*

When caring for patients with significant POI/POA with several previous failed cycles of ovulation induction, it is common to find women who do not respond at all to ovulation induction; they have no evidence of follicle growth and no estradiol rise. Paradoxically, we found that when we stop all medications and recheck in 3 days about half of such patients would show evidence of follicle growth and rising

Table 1 Comparison IVF parameters with early retrieval and standard retrieval among women with evidence of diminished ovarian reserve

IVF parameters	Early retrieval	Standard retrieval
Number of patients	24	13
Age (years)	39.4 ± 0.6	38.5 ± 0.6
Serum FSH (mIU/mL)	12.8 ± 1.3	11.3 ± 1.2
Serum AMH (mg/mL)	0.49 ± 0.09	0.43 ± 0.12
P4/E2 ratio on trigger day	2.49 ± 0.37	3.16 ± 0.68
Retrieved oocytes	3.4 ± 0.6	5.7 ± 1.3
Matured oocyte	2.7 ± 0.44	3.4 ± 0.9
% of mature oocytes	81.5 ± 4.5	55.8 ± 8.3[a]
Immature oocytes	0.45 ± 0.1	0.7 ± 0.2
% of immature oocytes	12.6 ± 3.4	14.4 ± 5.1
Atretic oocyte	0.32 ± 0.2	1.3 ± 0.3[a]
% of atretic oocyte	7.9 ± 3.0	28.2 ± 7.2[a]
Fertilized oocytes	2.2 ± 0.4	3.1 ± 0.7
% of fertilized oocytes	87.5 ± 5.2	86.8 ± 5.1
Total transferable embryos	1.6 ± 0.2	2.5 ± 0.3
High quality embryos	1.1 ± 0.2	0.9 ± 0.2
% of high quality embryos	68.2 ± 10.7	53.8 ± 9.3
Clinical pregnancy rate	41.7% (10/24)	7.7% (1/13)[a]

From Wu et al. Journal of Ovarian Research (2018) 11:23
[a]$P < 0.05$

estradiol. We have termed this paradoxical phenomenon "rebound." We now routinely ask patients to return for a "rebound check" 3–4 days after stopping ovulation induction. When we see evidence of such response, ovulation induction is restarted, and many of these patients reach retrieval.

Through August 2019, 49 women with maximal levels FSH greater than 20 mIU/mL, AMH less than 0.01 ng/mL, and failure to exhibit a rise in estradiol greater than 60 after more than 8 days of ovulation induction have been treated in "rebound" cycles in our practice. Of these 24 responded and ovulation induction was restarted. Twenty-two patients reached retrieval and 15 patients reached embryo transfer. Until now, managing the "rebound" has not resulted in a pregnancy.

6 Embryo Factors

6.1 *Fertilization and Implantation*

In vivo fertilization occurs in the fallopian tube within 24 h of ovulation. The fertilized zygote then travels down the fallopian tube over 3–4 days to the uterus, arriving there around the fifth day after ovulation. Implantation may not occur until 6–8 days following fertilization.

6.1.1 Fertilization

Fertilization is a complex process dependent on competent sperm being transported to the distal fallopian tube. Tubal disease that could hinder the ability of ovum pickup by the distal fimbria or hinder transport of either the oocyte, sperm, or fertilized zygote may all give rise to infertility. In the past tubal disease was surgically treated with various procedures designed to restore tubal patency. However, even in the best of hands, the live birth rate was often less than 25% within a year of surgery [111, 112]. Furthermore, after surgery to repair a damaged fallopian tube, the odds of ectopic pregnancy increase fourfold [113]. For these reasons, surgical approaches to tubal disease have fallen out of favor.

6.1.2 Ectopic Pregnancy

The incidence of ectopic pregnancy following IVF embryo transfer (ET) ranges from 1 to 2% [113–115]. Ectopic pregnancy following ET is more common among women with a history of tubal disease and less common following day-5 ET [115]. No one knows what happens to an embryo that has been transferred to the uterine cavity days before endometrial receptivity has been achieved. It may be that embryos move often back into the proximal fallopian tube, retracing the normal path of development. Since ectopic pregnancy is known to occur after ET, at least some embryos must migrate back into the fallopian tubes, but perhaps most do, and only a few unlucky embryos result in a tubal implantation. As noted above implantation will not begin for a few days after ET, so a day-3 ET will spend more time preimplantation than a day-5 embryo, increasing the risk of ectopic implantation for women with a history of tubal disease [114]. Women who used the contraceptive device known as Essure©, which creates proximal tubal occlusion, experienced lower pregnancy rates after IVF embryo transfer compared to those who were treated by laparoscopic salpingectomy before IVF [116]; perhaps the opportunity to migrate back into the fallopian tube improves the chance of a successful cycle? Thus, one may speculate that passage back to a normal tube may give embryos an advantage, while transit in a damaged tube creates a risk.

6.2 Embryo Selection

A typical cycle of in vitro fertilization will produce multiple oocytes and many embryos. As already noted above, the major rationale for using ovulation induction was to produce multiple oocytes and allow formation of multiple embryos. One goal of producing multiple embryos was to allow selection of the most favorable embryo or set of embryos for transfer. Over the years, various strategies have been used to select embryos and decide how many embryos to transfer.

6.2.1 Embryo Morphology

Once an egg becomes fertilized, the resulting zygote will begin to divide. Each cell division is an independent event based on each cell's individual metabolic response to its immediate environment. After 3 days in culture, we expect that a zygote will have divided three times, each time doubling the number of blastomeres. For this reason, we expect an embryo that has undergone three normal divisions to have eight blastomeres. Embryos with greater or fewer numbers of blastomeres might represent abnormal cell division and are considered less favorably. Embryos are also graded based on appearance color, texture, symmetry, and on the percent of small cytoplasmic fragments surrounding the blastomeres [117]. The best graded embryos are symmetrical and have few or no fragments (Table 2).

Embryos allowed to remain in culture for 5 days will, under normal conditions, progress to the blastocyst stage. The typical blastocyst will have a spherical trophectoderm made up of 200–300 cells and a much smaller inner cell mass. The trophectoderm will develop into the placenta, and the inner cell mass will go on to form the embryo proper. Day-5 embryos are scored based on their stage of development and on the characteristics of the cells in the inner cell mass and in the trophectoderm [117] (Table 2). Since the process of embryo implantation does not occur until several days after fertilization, transfers could in theory occur anytime in the first 6 days after fertilization. When embryo culture methods had improved enough to allow culture of embryos to blastocyst, it soon became apparent that embryos which had survived to the blastocyst stage had a greater chance of implanting and establishing a pregnancy that could result in a live birth. Although many assumed that culture to blastocyst resulted in a more successful embryo, this was not the case. Embryos that could survive in the laboratory to the blastocyst stage simply proved that they were stronger, not as a result of extended culture but because they had always been the most fit of their cohort. One of the costs of using extended culture to identify highly successful embryos is the loss of embryos that could not survive in extended culture. Current best evidence suggests that while blastocyst culture allows selection of a successful embryo for a fresh embryo transfer, because fewer embryos are cryopreserved, there is no evidence of difference in cumulative pregnancy rates using embryos produced from a single oocyte retrieval [118].

Table 2 SART grading system

Growth phase	Overall grade	Stage
Cleavage	Good, fair, poor	Cell #: 1 through >8 Fragmentation: 0%, <10%, 11–25%, >25% Symmetry: perfect, moderately asymmetric, severely asymmetric
Morula	Good, fair, poor	Compaction: complete, incomplete Fragmentation: 0%, <10%, 11–25%, >25%
Blastocyst	Good, fair, poor	Expansion: early, expanding, expanded, hatched Inner cell mass: good, fair, poor Trophectoderm: good, fair, poor

From J Assist Reprod Genet (2010) 27:437–439

6.2.2 Preimplantation Genetic Testing

In the 1980s preimplantation genetic testing (PGT) was developed with the goal of identifying genetic disease when both parents were known to be carriers for conditions like cystic fibrosis, Huntington's disease, or hemophilia. Techniques were soon extended to try to rule out balanced translocations and aneuploidies in embryos before embryo transfer.

This technique, first called preimplantation genetic diagnosis (PGD), used fluorescence in situ hybridization (FISH) to identify aneuploidy in polar bodies or single blastomere biopsies from day-3 embryos [119–121]. As evidence accumulated over time, it became clear that damage to the embryo from blastomere biopsy and the inaccuracy of the FISH technique [122] actually decreased the chance of a successful pregnancy [123–125].

In response to these observations, new techniques were developed to test embryos at a later stage of development when more cells could be sampled recognizing that at this later stage of development these cells would represent a smaller percentage of the resulting embryo and hopefully lead to less embryo damage [126, 127]. The resulting technique of trophectoderm biopsy would sample 4 to 6 cells from the trophectoderm and would use new methods of genetic analysis of these cells that would allow reporting of the ploidy of all 24 chromosomes [128–130].

For young women less than 35 years old, selection of a blastocyst with a euploid biopsy promised an excellent chance of a successful pregnancy. However, by the age 40 years, almost 60% of embryos had aneuploid biopsy results, while by 44 years the percentage of aneuploid biopsies increased to 88% and more than 40% of couples had no embryos with euploid biopsy for transfer [131].

Recognizing that no test is 100% accurate, we and others began offering to transfer embryos that had been called "aneuploid" based on their trophectoderm biopsy. We realized that the only way to lose all chance of a successful pregnancy was to never offer an embryo transfer. When these embryos were transferred, it turned out that a substantial number were able to achieve pregnancy and normal live birth [132, 133]. A recent survey found more than 400 live births after transfer of embryos determined by PGT to be abnormal [134]. It turned out that the accuracy of preimplantation testing was limited by the mosaic nature of early human embryos [135] and by the ability of some embryos to self-correct mitotically derived aneuploidy [136, 137]. Today, preimplantation genetic testing (PGT) is widely practiced, though many still consider it to be controversial [138]. In general, we do not recommend PGT to our patients with diminished ovarian reserve as we believe our role is to promote the best chance of pregnancy and not to try to guarantee a so-called perfect embryo.

References

1. Brugh MV, Lipshultz L. Male factor infertility: evaluation and management. Med Clin North Am. 2004;88(2):367–85.
2. Faddy MJ, Gosden RG, Gougeon A, Richardson SJ, Nelson JF. Accelerated disappearance of ovarian follicles in mid-life: implications for forecasting menopause. Hum Reprod. 1992;7(10):1342–6.
3. Iliodromiti S, Nelson SM. Biomarkers of ovarian reserve. Biomark Med. 2013;7(1):147–58.
4. Coelho Neto MA, Ludwin A, Borrell A, Benacerraf B, Dewailly D, da Silva Costa F, Condous G, Alcazar JL, Jokubkiene L, Guerriero S, Van den Bosch T, Martins WP. Counting ovarian antral follicles by ultrasound: a practical guide. Ultrasound Obstet Gynecol. 2018;51(1):10–20.
5. Hendriks DJ, Kwee J, Mol BW, te Velde ER, Broekmans FJ. Ultrasonography as a tool for the prediction of outcome in IVF patients: a comparative meta-analysis of ovarian volume and antral follicle count. Fertil Steril. 2007;87(4):764–75.
6. Gibreel A, Maheshwari A, Bhattacharya S, Johnson NP. Ultrasound tests of ovarian reserve; a systematic review of accuracy in predicting fertility outcomes. Hum Fertil (Camb). 2009;12(2):95–106.
7. Broer SL, Dolleman M, Opmeer BC, Fauser BC, Mol BW, Broekmans FJ. AMH and AFC as predictors of excessive response in controlled ovarian hyperstimulation: a meta-analysis. Hum Reprod Update. 2011;17(1):46–54.
8. Scott RT, Toner JP, Muasher SJ, Oehninger S, Robinson S, Rosenwaks Z. Follicle-stimulating hormone levels on cycle day 3 are predictive of in vitro fertilization outcome. Fertil Steril. 1989;51(4):651–4.
9. Toner JP. The significance of elevated FSH for reproductive function. Baillieres Clin Obstet Gynaecol. 1993;7(2):283–95.
10. Toner JP, Philput CB, Jones GS, Muasher SJ. Basal follicle-stimulating hormone level is a better predictor of in vitro fertilization performance than age. Fertil Steril. 1991;55(4):784–91.
11. Ling N, DePaolo LV, Bicsak TA, Shimasaki S. Novel ovarian regulatory peptides: inhibin, activin, and follistatin. Clin Obstet Gynecol. 1990;33(3):690–702.
12. Kligman I, Rosenwaks Z. Differentiating clinical profiles: predicting good responders, poor responders, and hyperresponders. Fertil Steril. 2001;76(6):1185–90.
13. Gingold JA, Lee JA, Whitehouse MC, Rodriguez-Purata J, Sandler B, Grunfeld L, Mukherjee T, Copperman AB. Maximum basal FSH predicts reproductive outcome better than cycle-specific basal FSH levels: waiting for a "better" month conveys limited retrieval benefits. Reprod Biol Endocrinol. 2015;13:91.
14. Lass A, Gerrard A, Abusheikha N, Akagbosu F, Brinsden P. IVF performance of women who have fluctuating early follicular FSH levels. J Assist Reprod Genet. 2000;17(10):566–73.
15. Barad DH, Weghofer A, Gleicher N. Age-specific levels for basal follicle-stimulating hormone assessment of ovarian function. Obstet Gynecol. 2007b;109(6):1404–10.
16. Fang T, Su Z, Wang L, Yuan P, Li R, Ouyang N, Zheng L, Wang W. Predictive value of age-specific FSH levels for IVF-ET outcome in women with normal ovarian function. Reprod Biol Endocrinol. 2015;13:63.
17. Fasouliotis SJ, Simon A, Laufer N. Evaluation and treatment of low responders in assisted reproductive technology: a challenge to meet. J Assist Reprod Genet. 2000;17(7):357–73.
18. Gleicher N, Barad D. "Ovarian age-based" stimulation of young women with diminished ovarian reserve results in excellent pregnancy rates with in vitro fertilization. Fertil Steril. 2006;86(6):1621–5.
19. Toner JP, Flood JT. Fertility after the age of 40. Obstet Gynecol Clin N Am. 1993;20(2):261–72.
20. Kushnir VA, Safdie M, Darmon SK, Albertini DF, Barad DH, Gleicher N. Age-specific IVF outcomes in infertile women with baseline FSH levels >/=20 mIU/mL. Reprod Sci. 2018;25(6):893–8.

21. Barad DH, Weghofer A, Gleicher N. Comparing anti-Mullerian hormone (AMH) and follicle-stimulating hormone (FSH) as predictors of ovarian function. Fertil Steril. 2009;91(4 Suppl):1553–5.
22. Barad DH, Weghofer A, Gleicher N. Utility of age-specific serum anti-Mullerian hormone concentrations. Reprod Biomed Online. 2011;22(3):284–91.
23. Gleicher N, Darmon SK, Kushnir VA, Weghofer A, Wang Q, Zhang L, Albertini DF, Barad DH. How FSH and AMH reflect probabilities of oocyte numbers in poor prognosis patients with small oocyte yields. Endocrine. 2016a;54(2):476–83.
24. Gleicher N, Weghofer A, Barad DH. Anti-Mullerian hormone (AMH) defines, independent of age, low versus good live-birth chances in women with severely diminished ovarian reserve. Fertil Steril. 2010;94(7):2824–7.
25. Kushnir VA, Seifer DB, Barad DH, Sen A, Gleicher N. Potential therapeutic applications of human anti-Mullerian hormone (AMH) analogues in reproductive medicine. J Assist Reprod Genet. 2017;34(9):1105–13.
26. Barad DH, Kim A, Kubba H, Weghofer A, Gleicher N. Does hormonal contraception prior to in vitro fertilization (IVF) negatively affect oocyte yields? A pilot study. Reprod Biol Endocrinol. 2013;11:28.
27. Weghofer A, Dietrich W, Ortner I, Bieglmayer C, Barad D, Gleicher N. Anti-Mullerian hormone levels decline under hormonal suppression: a prospective analysis in fertile women after delivery. Reprod Biol Endocrinol. 2011;9:98.
28. Hiedar Z, Bakhtiyari M, Foroozanfard F, Mirzamoradi M. Age-specific reference values and cut-off points for anti-mullerian hormone in infertile women following a long agonist treatment protocol for IVF. J Endocrinol Investig. 2018;41(7):773–80.
29. Seifer DB, Baker VL, Leader B. Age-specific serum anti-Mullerian hormone values for 17,120 women presenting to fertility centers within the United States. Fertil Steril. 2011;95(2):747–50.
30. Steptoe PC, Edwards RG. Birth after the reimplantation of a human embryo. Lancet. 1978;2(8085):366.
31. Fleming R, Coutts JR. Induction of multiple follicular development for IVF. Br Med Bull. 1990;46(3):596–615.
32. Fauser BC, Devroey P, Macklon NS. Multiple birth resulting from ovarian stimulation for subfertility treatment. Lancet. 2005;365(9473):1807–16.
33. Hamoda H, Sunkara S, Khalaf Y, Braude P, El-Toukhy T. Outcome of fresh IVF/ICSI cycles in relation to the number of oocytes collected: a review of 4,701 treatment cycles. Hum Reprod. 2010;25.
34. Magnusson Å, Källen K, Thurin-Kjellberg A, Bergh C. The number of oocytes retrieved during IVF: a balance between efficacy and safety. Hum Reprod. 2017;33(1):58–64.
35. van der Gaast MH, Eijkemans MJ, van der Net JB, de Boer EJ, Burger CW, van Leeuwen FE, Fauser BC, Macklon NS. Optimum number of oocytes for a successful first IVF treatment cycle. Reprod Biomed Online. 2006;13(4):476–80.
36. Stanger JD, Yovich JL. Follicle recruitment determines IVF productivity rate via the number of embryos frozen and subsequent transfers. Reprod Biomed Online. 2013;27(3):286–96.
37. Arce JC, Andersen AN, Fernandez-Sanchez M, Visnova H, Bosch E, Garcia-Velasco JA, Barri P, de Sutter P, Klein BM, Fauser BC. Ovarian response to recombinant human follicle-stimulating hormone: a randomized, antimullerian hormone-stratified, dose-response trial in women undergoing in vitro fertilization/intracytoplasmic sperm injection. Fertil Steril. 2014;102(6):1633–40.e1635.
38. Lekamge DN, Lane M, Gilchrist RB, Tremellen KP. Increased gonadotrophin stimulation does not improve IVF outcomes in patients with predicted poor ovarian reserve. J Assist Reprod Genet. 2008;25(11–12):515–21.
39. Out HJ, Braat DD, Lintsen BM, Gurgan T, Bukulmez O, Gokmen O, Keles G, Caballero P, Gonzalez JM, Fabregues F, Balasch J, Roulier R. Increasing the daily dose of recombinant

follicle stimulating hormone (Puregon) does not compensate for the age-related decline in retrievable oocytes after ovarian stimulation. Hum Reprod. 2000;15(1):29–35.

40. Rustamov O, Wilkinson J, La Marca A, Fitzgerald C, Roberts S. How much variation in oocyte yield after controlled ovarian stimulation can be explained? A multilevel modelling study. Human Reproduction Open. 2017;2017:hox018.
41. Kawwass JF, Hipp HS, Session DR, Kissin DM, Jamieson DJ, A. R. T. S. S. G. National. Severity of diminished ovarian reserve and chance of success with assisted reproductive technology. J Reprod Med. 2017;62(3–4):153–60.
42. Lensen SF, Wilkinson J, Leijdekkers JA, La Marca A, Mol BWJ, Marjoribanks J, Torrance H, Broekmans FJ. Individualised gonadotropin dose selection using markers of ovarian reserve for women undergoing in vitro fertilisation plus intracytoplasmic sperm injection (IVF/ICSI). Cochrane Database Syst Rev. 2018;2:CD012693.
43. Almog B, Shehata F, Shalom-Paz E, Tan SL, Tulandi T. Age-related normogram for antral follicle count: McGill reference guide. Fertil Steril. 2011;95(2):663–6.
44. Holte J, Brodin T, Berglund L, Hadziosmanovic N, Olovsson M, Bergh T. Antral follicle counts are strongly associated with live-birth rates after assisted reproduction, with superior treatment outcome in women with polycystic ovaries. Fertil Steril. 2011;96(3):594–9.
45. Hsu A, Arny M, Knee AB, Bell C, Cook E, Novak AL, Grow DR. Antral follicle count in clinical practice: analyzing clinical relevance. Fertil Steril. 2011;95(2):474–9.
46. Muasher SJ, Abdallah RT, Hubayter ZR. Optimal stimulation protocols for in vitro fertilization. Fertil Steril. 2006;86(2):267–73.
47. Longcope C. Adrenal and gonadal androgen secretion in normal females. Clin Endocrinol Metab. 1986;15(2):213–28.
48. Endoh A, Kristiansen SB, Casson PR, Buster JE, Hornsby PJ. The zona reticularis is the site of biosynthesis of dehydroepiandrosterone and dehydroepiandrosterone sulfate in the adult human adrenal cortex resulting from its low expression of 3 beta-hydroxysteroid dehydrogenase. J Clin Endocrinol Metab. 1996;81(10):3558–65.
49. Hornsby PJ. Biosynthesis of DHEAS by the human adrenal cortex and its age-related decline. Ann N Y Acad Sci. 1995;774:29–46.
50. Hornsby PJ. Aging of the human adrenal cortex. Sci Aging Knowl Environ. 2004;2004(35):re6.
51. McNatty KP, Makris A, De Grazia C, Osathanondh R, Ryan KJ. The production of progesterone, androgens and oestrogens by human granulosa cells in vitro and in vivo. J Steroid Biochem. 1979;11(1C):775–9.
52. Ryan KJ. Granulosa-thecal cell interaction in ovarian steroidogenesis. J Steroid Biochem. 1979;11(1C):799–800.
53. Prizant H, Gleicher N, Sen A. Androgen actions in the ovary: balance is key. J Endocrinol. 2014;222(3):R141–51.
54. Sen A, Hammes SR. Granulosa cell-specific androgen receptors are critical regulators of ovarian development and function. Mol Endocrinol. 2010;24(7):1393–403.
55. Sen A, Prizant H, Light A, Biswas A, Hayes E, Lee HJ, Barad D, Gleicher N, Hammes SR. Androgens regulate ovarian follicular development by increasing follicle stimulating hormone receptor and microRNA-125b expression. Proc Natl Acad Sci U S A. 2014;111(8):3008–13.
56. Sen A, Prizant H, Hammes SR. Understanding extranuclear (nongenomic) androgen signaling: what a frog oocyte can tell us about human biology. Steroids. 2011;76(9):822–8.
57. Barad DH, Gleicher N. Increased oocyte production after treatment with dehydroepiandrosterone. Fertil Steril. 2005;84(3):756.
58. Casson PR, Lindsay MS, Pisarska MD, Carson SA, Buster JE. Dehydroepiandrosterone supplementation augments ovarian stimulation in poor responders: a case series. Hum Reprod. 2000;15(10):2129–32.
59. Barad D, Brill H, Gleicher N. Update on the use of dehydroepiandrosterone supplementation among women with diminished ovarian function. J Assist Reprod Genet. 2007a;24(12):629–34.

60. Barad D, Gleicher N. Effect of dehydroepiandrosterone on oocyte and embryo yields, embryo grade and cell number in IVF. Hum Reprod. 2006;21(11):2845–9.
61. Liu Y, Hu L, Fan L, Wang F. Efficacy of dehydroepiandrosterone (DHEA) supplementation for in vitro fertilization and embryo transfer cycles: a systematic review and meta-analysis. Gynecol Endocrinol. 2018;34(3):178–83.
62. Nagels HE, Rishworth JR, Siristatidis CS, Kroon B. Androgens (dehydroepiandrosterone or testosterone) for women undergoing assisted reproduction. Cochrane Database Syst Rev. 2015;11:CD009749.
63. Narkwichean A, Maalouf W, Baumgarten M, Polanski L, Raine-Fenning N, Campbell B, Jayaprakasan K. Efficacy of dehydroepiandrosterone (DHEA) to overcome the effect of ovarian ageing (DITTO): a proof of principle double blinded randomized placebo controlled trial. Eur J Obstet Gynecol Reprod Biol. 2017;218:39–48.
64. Griesinger G, Venetis CA, Tarlatzis B, Kolibianakis EM. To pill or not to pill in GnRH-antagonist cycles: the answer is in the data already! Reprod Biomed Online. 2015;31(1):6–8.
65. Deb S, Campbell BK, Pincott-Allen C, Clewes JS, Cumberpatch G, Raine-Fenning NJ. Quantifying effect of combined oral contraceptive pill on functional ovarian reserve as measured by serum anti-Mullerian hormone and small antral follicle count using three-dimensional ultrasound. Ultrasound Obstet Gynecol. 2012;39(5):574–80.
66. Gleicher N, Kim A, Weghofer A, Shohat-Tal A, Lazzaroni E, Lee HJ, Barad DH. Starting and resulting testosterone levels after androgen supplementation determine at all ages in vitro fertilization (IVF) pregnancy rates in women with diminished ovarian reserve (DOR). J Assist Reprod Genet. 2013;30(1):49–62.
67. Abir R, Garor R, Felz C, Nitke S, Krissi H, Fisch B. Growth hormone and its receptor in human ovaries from fetuses and adults. Fertil Steril. 2008;90(4 Suppl):1333–9.
68. Buyalos RP. Insulin-like growth factors: clinical experience in ovarian function. Am J Med. 1995;98(1A):55S–66S.
69. Menezo YJ, el Mouatassim S, Chavrier M, Servy EJ, Nicolet B. Human oocytes and preimplantation embryos express mRNA for growth hormone receptor. Zygote. 2003;11(4):293–7.
70. Zhou P, Baumgarten SC, Wu Y, Bennett J, Winston N, Hirshfeld-Cytron J, Stocco C. IGF-I signaling is essential for FSH stimulation of AKT and steroidogenic genes in granulosa cells. Mol Endocrinol. 2013;27(3):511–23.
71. Baker J, Hardy MP, Zhou J, Bondy C, Lupu F, Bellve AR, Efstratiadis A. Effects of an Igf1 gene null mutation on mouse reproduction. Mol Endocrinol. 1996;10(7):903–18.
72. Zhou J, Kumar TR, Matzuk MM, Bondy C. Insulin-like growth factor I regulates gonadotropin responsiveness in the murine ovary. Mol Endocrinol. 1997;11(13):1924–33.
73. Chun SY, Billig H, Tilly JL, Furuta I, Tsafriri A, Hsueh AJ. Gonadotropin suppression of apoptosis in cultured preovulatory follicles: mediatory role of endogenous insulin-like growth factor I. Endocrinology. 1994;135(5):1845–53.
74. Adashi EY, Resnick CE, D'Ercole AJ, Svoboda ME, van Wyk JJ. Insulin-like growth factors as intraovarian regulators of granulosa cell growth and function*. Endocr Rev. 1985;6(3):400–20.
75. Oosterhuis GJ, Vermes I, Lambalk CB, Michgelsen HW, Schoemaker J. Insulin-like growth factor (IGF)-I and IGF binding protein-3 concentrations in fluid from human stimulated follicles. Hum Reprod. 1998;13(2):285–9.
76. Regan SLP, Knight PG, Yovich JL, Arfuso F, Dharmarajan A. Growth hormone during in vitro fertilization in older women modulates the density of receptors in granulosa cells, with improved pregnancy outcomes. Fertil Steril. 2018;110(7):1298–310.
77. Bergh C, Hillensjo T, Wikland M, Nilsson L, Borg G, Hamberger L. Adjuvant growth hormone treatment during in vitro fertilization: a randomized, placebo-controlled study. Fertil Steril. 1994;62(1):113–20.
78. Hazout A, Junca A, Menezo Y, Demouzon J, Cohen-Bacrie P. Effect of growth hormone on oocyte competence in patients with multiple IVF failures. Reprod Biomed Online. 2009;18(5):664–70.

79. Kucuk T, Kozinoglu H, Kaba A. Growth hormone co-treatment within a GnRH agonist long protocol in patients with poor ovarian response: a prospective, randomized, clinical trial. J Assist Reprod Genet. 2008;25(4):123–7.
80. Owen EJ, West C, Mason BA, Jacobs HS. Co-treatment with growth hormone of sub-optimal responders in IVF-ET. Hum Reprod. 1991;6(4):524–8.
81. Suikkari A, MacLachlan V, Koistinen R, Seppala M, Healy D. Double-blind placebo controlled study: human biosynthetic growth hormone for assisted reproductive technology. Fertil Steril. 1996;65(4):800–5.
82. Tesarik J, Hazout A, Mendoza C. Improvement of delivery and live birth rates after ICSI in women aged >40 years by ovarian co-stimulation with growth hormone. Hum Reprod. 2005;20(9):2536–41.
83. Zhuang GL, Wong SX, Zhou CQ. [The effect of co-administration of low dosage growth hormone and gonadotropin for ovarian hyperstimulation in vitro fertilization and embryo transfer]. Zhonghua Fu Chan Ke Za Zhi. 1994;29(8):471–74, 510.
84. Dakhly DMR, Bassiouny YA, Bayoumi YA, Hassan MA, Gouda HM, Hassan AA. The addition of growth hormone adjuvant therapy to the long down regulation protocol in poor responders undergoing in vitro fertilization: randomized control trial. Eur J Obstet Gynecol Reprod Biol. 2018;228:161–5.
85. Norman RJ, Alvino H, Hull LM, Mol BW, Hart RJ, Kelly TL, Rombauts L, investigators L. Human growth hormone for poor responders: a randomized placebo-controlled trial provides no evidence for improved live birth rate. Reprod Biomed Online. 2019;38(6):908–15.
86. Casson PR, Santoro N, Elkind-Hirsch K, Carson SA, Hornsby PJ, Abraham G, Buster JE. Postmenopausal dehydroepiandrosterone administration increases free insulin-like growth factor-I and decreases high-density lipoprotein: a six-month trial. Fertil Steril. 1998;70(1):107–10.
87. Yoshimura Y, Ando M, Nagamatsu S, Iwashita M, Adachi T, Sueoka K, Miyazaki T, Kuji N, Tanaka M. Effects of insulin-like growth factor-I on follicle growth, oocyte maturation, and ovarian steroidogenesis and plasminogen activator activity in the rabbit. Biol Reprod. 1996a;55(1):152–60.
88. Yoshimura Y, Aoki N, Sueoka K, Miyazaki T, Kuji N, Tanaka M, Kobayashi T. Interactions between insulin-like growth factor-I (IGF-I) and the renin-angiotensin system in follicular growth and ovulation. J Clin Invest. 1996b;98(2):308–16.
89. Pantos K, Nitsos N, Kokkali G, Vaxevanoglou T, Markomichali C, Pantou A, Grammatis M, Lazaros L, Sfakianoudis K. Ovarian rejuvenation and folliculogenesis reactivation in perimenopausal women after autologous platelet-rich plasma treatment ESHRE 32nd Annual Meeting. Helsinki, Finland. Hum Reprod: i301; 2016.
90. Fabi S, Sundaram H. The potential of topical and injectable growth factors and cytokines for skin rejuvenation. Facial Plast Surg. 2014;30(02):157–71.
91. Xie X, Zhang C, Tuan RS. Biology of platelet-rich plasma and its clinical application in cartilage repair. Arthritis Res Ther. 2014;16(1):204.
92. Macaulay IC, Carr P, Gusnanto A, Ouwehand WH, Fitzgerald D, Watkins NA. Platelet genomics and proteomics in human health and disease. J Clin Invest. 2005;115:3370.
93. McRedmond JP, Park SD, Reilly DF, Coppinger JA, Maguire PB, Shields DC, Fitzgerald DJ. Integration of proteomics and genomics in platelets: a profile of platelet proteins and platelet-specific genes. Mol Cell Proteomics. 2004;3:133.
94. Watson SP, Bahou WF, Fitzgerald D, Ouwehand W, Rao AK, Leavitt AD. ISTH platelet physiology subcommittee: mapping the platelet proteome: a report of the ISTH platelet physiology subcommittee. J Thromb Haemost. 2005;3:2098.
95. Sills ES, Wood SH. Autologous activated platelet-rich plasma injection into adult human ovary tissue: molecular mechanism, analysis, and discussion of reproductive response. Biosci Rep, 2019;39(6).

96. Farimani M, Heshmati S, Poorolajal J, Bahmanzadeh M. A report on three live births in women with poor ovarian response following intra-ovarian injection of platelet-rich plasma (PRP). Mol Biol Rep. 2019;46(2):1611–6.
97. Hosseini L, Shirazi A, Naderi MM, Shams-Esfandabadi N, Borjian Boroujeni S, Sarvari A, Sadeghnia S, Behzadi B, Akhondi MM. Platelet-rich plasma promotes the development of isolated human primordial and primary follicles to the preantral stage. Reprod Biomed Online. 2017;35(4):343–50.
98. Sills ES, Rickers NS, Li X, Palermo GD. First data on in vitro fertilization and blastocyst formation after intraovarian injection of calcium gluconate-activated autologous platelet rich plasma. Gynecol Endocrinol. 2018;34(9):756–60.
99. Pantos K, Simopoulou M, Pantou A, Rapani A, Tsioulou P, Nitsos N, Syrkos S, Pappas A, Koutsilieris M, Sfakianoudis K. A case series on natural conceptions resulting in ongoing pregnancies in menopausal and prematurely menopausal women following platelet-rich plasma treatment. Cell Transplant. 2019;28(9–10):1333–40. https://doi.org/10.1177/0963689719859539.
100. Wu YG, Barad DH, Kushnir VA, Wang Q, Zhang L, Darmon SK, Albertini DF, Gleicher N. With low ovarian reserve, highly individualized egg retrieval (HIER) improves IVF results by avoiding premature luteinization. J Ovarian Res. 2018;11(1):23.
101. Navot D, Bergh PA, Williams MA, Garrisi GJ, Guzman I, Sandler B, Grunfeld L. Poor oocyte quality rather than implantation failure as a cause of age-related decline in female fertility. Lancet. 1991;337(8754):1375–7.
102. Wu YG, Barad DH, Kushnir VA, Lazzaroni E, Wang Q, Albertini DF, Gleicher N. Aging-related premature luteinization of granulosa cells is avoided by early oocyte retrieval. J Endocrinol. 2015;226(3):167–80.
103. Da Broi MG, Giorgi VSI, Wang F, Keefe DL, Albertini D, Navarro PA. Influence of follicular fluid and cumulus cells on oocyte quality: clinical implications. J Assist Reprod Genet. 2018;35(5):735–51.
104. Herlands RL, Schultz RM. Regulation of mouse oocyte growth: probable nutritional role for intercellular communication between follicle cells and oocytes in oocyte growth. J Exp Zool. 1984;229(2):317–25.
105. Viveiros MM, De La Fuente R. Chapter 11—regulation of mammalian oocyte maturation. In: Leung PCK, Adashi EY, editors. The ovary. 3rd ed: Academic Press; 2019. p. 165–80.
106. Seifer DB, Charland C, Berlinsky D, Penzias AS, Haning RV Jr, Naftolin F, Barker BE. Proliferative index of human luteinized granulosa cells varies as a function of ovarian reserve. Am J Obstet Gynecol. 1993;169(6):1531–5.
107. Seifer DB, Gardiner AC, Ferreira KA, Peluso JJ. Apoptosis as a function of ovarian reserve in women undergoing in vitro fertilization. Fertil Steril. 1996;66(4):593–8.
108. Barad DH. Infertility surgery by laparotomy. Curr Opin Obstet Gynecol. 1991;3(3):398–403.
109. Teoh TG, Kondaveeti U, Darling MR. The management of female infertility by tubal microsurgical reconstruction: a ten year review. Ir J Med Sci. 1995;164(3):212–4.
110. Farquhar CM. Ectopic pregnancy. Lancet. 2005;366(9485):583–91.
111. Johnson N, van Voorst S, Sowter MC, Strandell A, Mol BW. Surgical treatment for tubal disease in women due to undergo in vitro fertilisation. Cochrane Database Syst Rev. 2010;(1):CD002125.
112. Tsiami A, Chaimani A, Mavridis D, Siskou M, Assimakopoulos E, Sotiriadis A. Surgical treatment for hydrosalpinx prior to in-vitro fertilization embryo transfer: a network meta-analysis. Ultrasound Obstet Gynecol. 2016;48(4):434–45.
113. Pereira N, Pryor KP, Voskuilen-Gonzalez A, Lekovich JP, Elias RT, Spandorfer SD, Rosenwaks Z. Ovarian response and in vitro fertilization outcomes after salpingectomy: does salpingectomy indication matter? J Minim Invasive Gynecol. 2017;24(3):446–54.e441.
114. Li Z, Sullivan EA, Chapman M, Farquhar C, Wang YA. Risk of ectopic pregnancy lowest with transfer of single frozen blastocyst. Hum Reprod. 2015;30(9):2048–54.

115. Santos-Ribeiro S, Tournaye H, Polyzos NP. Trends in ectopic pregnancy rates following assisted reproductive technologies in the UK: a 12-year nationwide analysis including 160 000 pregnancies. Hum Reprod. 2016;31(2):393–402.
116. Xu B, Zhang Q, Zhao J, Wang Y, Xu D, Li Y. Pregnancy outcome of in vitro fertilization after Essure and laparoscopic management of hydrosalpinx: a systematic review and meta-analysis. Fertil Steril. 2017;108(1):84–95.e85.
117. Racowsky C, Vernon M, Mayer J, Ball GD, Behr B, Pomeroy KO, Wininger D, Gibbons W, Conaghan J, Stern JE. Standardization of grading embryo morphology. J Assist Reprod Genet. 2010;27(8):437–9.
118. Glujovsky D, Farquhar C, Quinteiro Retamar AM, Alvarez Sedo CR, Blake D. Cleavage stage versus blastocyst stage embryo transfer in assisted reproductive technology. Cochrane Database Syst Rev. 2016;6:CD002118.
119. Kuliev A, Verlinsky Y. Place of preimplantation diagnosis in genetic practice. Am J Med Genet A. 2005;134A(1):105–10.
120. Márquez C, Sandalinas M, Bahçe M, Al ikani M, Munné S. Chromosome abnormalities in 1255 cleavage-stage human embryos. Reprod Biomed Online. 2000;1(1):17–26.
121. Munné S, Alikani M, Tomkin G, Grifo J, Cohen J. Embryo morphology, developmental rates, and maternal age are correlated with chromosome abnormalities**Presented at the 50th Annual Meeting of The American Fertility Society, San Antonio, Texas, November 4 to 9, 1994, where it was awarded the prize paper of the Society for Assisted Reproductive Technology. Fertil Steril. 1995;64(2):382–91.
122. Northrop LE, Treff NR, Levy B, Scott RT Jr. SNP microarray-based 24 chromosome aneuploidy screening demonstrates that cleavage-stage FISH poorly predicts aneuploidy in embryos that develop to morphologically normal blastocysts. Mol Hum Reprod. 2010;16(8):590–600.
123. Gleicher N, Kushnir VA, Barad DH. Preimplantation genetic screening (PGS) still in search of a clinical application: a systematic review. Reprod Biol Endocrinol. 2014;12(1):22.
124. Hardarson T, Hanson C, Lundin K, Hillensjo T, Nilsson L, Stevic J, Reismer E, Borg K, Wikland M, Bergh C. Preimplantation genetic screening in women of advanced maternal age caused a decrease in clinical pregnancy rate: a randomized controlled trial. Hum Reprod. 2008;23(12):2806–12.
125. Mastenbroek S, Twisk M, van der Veen F, Repping S. Preimplantation genetic screening: a systematic review and meta-analysis of RCTs. Hum Reprod Update. 2011;17(4):454–66.
126. de Boer KA, Catt JW, Jansen RP, Leigh D, McArthur S. Moving to blastocyst biopsy for preimplantation genetic diagnosis and single embryo transfer at Sydney IVF. Fertil Steril. 2004;82(2):295–8.
127. McArthur SJ, Leigh D, Marshall JT, de Boer KA, Jansen RP. Pregnancies and live births after trophectoderm biopsy and preimplantation genetic testing of human blastocysts. Fertil Steril. 2005;84(6):1628–36.
128. Marin D, Zimmerman R, Tao X, Zhan Y, Scott RT Jr, Treff NR. Validation of a targeted next generation sequencing-based comprehensive chromosome screening platform for detection of triploidy in human blastocysts. Reprod Biomed Online. 2018;36(4):388–95.
129. Scott RT Jr, Ferry K, Su J, Tao X, Scott K, Treff NR. Comprehensive chromosome screening is highly predictive of the reproductive potential of human embryos: a prospective, blinded, nonselection study. Fertil Steril. 2012;97(4):870–5.
130. Treff NR, Forman EJ, Scott RT Jr. Next-generation sequencing for preimplantation genetic diagnosis. Fertil Steril. 2013;99(6):e17–8.
131. Franasiak JM, Forman EJ, Hong KH, Werner MD, Upham KM, Treff NR, Scott RT Jr. The nature of aneuploidy with increasing age of the female partner: a review of 15,169 consecutive trophectoderm biopsies evaluated with comprehensive chromosomal screening. Fertil Steril. 2014;101(3):656–63.. e651
132. Gleicher N, Vidali A, Braverman J, Kushnir VA, Barad DH, Hudson C, Wu YG, Wang Q, Zhang L, Albertini DF, P. G. S. C. S. G. International. Accuracy of preimplantation genetic

screening (PGS) is compromised by degree of mosaicism of human embryos. Reprod Biol Endocrinol. 2016b;14(1):54.
133. Greco E, Minasi MG, Fiorentino F. Healthy babies after intrauterine transfer of mosaic aneuploid blastocysts. N Engl J Med. 2015;373(21):2089–90.
134. Patrizio P, Shoham G, Shoham Z, Leong M, Barad DH, Gleicher N. Worldwide live births following the transfer of chromosomally "abnormal" embryos after PGT/A: results of a worldwide web-based survey. J Assist Reprod Genet. 2019;36:1599.
135. Tiegs AW, Hodes-Wertz B, McCulloh DH, Munne S, Grifo JA. Discrepant diagnosis rate of array comparative genomic hybridization in thawed euploid blastocysts. J Assist Reprod Genet. 2016;33(7):893–7.
136. Bolton H, Graham SJL, Van der Aa N, Kumar P, Theunis K, Fernandez Gallardo E, Voet T, Zernicka-Goetz M. Mouse model of chromosome mosaicism reveals lineage-specific depletion of aneuploid cells and normal developmental potential. Nat Commun. 2016;7:11165.
137. Santos MA, Teklenburg G, Macklon NS, Van Opstal D, Schuring-Blom GH, Krijtenburg PJ, de Vreeden-Elbertse J, Fauser BC, Baart EB. The fate of the mosaic embryo: chromosomal constitution and development of day 4, 5 and 8 human embryos. Hum Reprod. 2010;25(8):1916–26.
138. Takahashi S, Patrizio P. The impact of mosaic embryos on procreative liberty and procreative responsibility: time to put innovative technology on "pause". Curr Stem Cell Rep. 2019;5:125.

Role of Hormones in Common Benign Uterine Lesions: Endometrial Polyps, Leiomyomas, and Adenomyosis

Myriam Kossaï and Frédérique Penault-Llorca

1 Introduction

Leiomyoma, adenomyosis, and endometrial polyps are benign uterine neoplasms or disorders. They are considered a specific entity in the PALM-COEIN FIGO [1]. They are absent before menarche and regress rapidly after menopause, indicating that sex steroid hormones (estrogen and progesterone) play a pivotal role in the development of these diseases. Estrogen and progesterone are secreted mainly by the ovaries and in smaller amounts by the adrenal glands. They are secreted cyclically during the reproductive life and are required for the process of implantation, which is the result of a series of complex interactions between the decidualized endometrium and the early embryo [2].

Leiomyoma, adenomyosis, and endometrial polyps seem to develop in the context of hormonal imbalances, in association with various factors ranging from genetic factors to modifiable lifestyle factors. In this chapter we define these entities and describe our current knowledge regarding their etiopathogenesis and the influence of sex steroid hormones on their development. Available and emerging therapy is presented for each disease.

M. Kossaï (✉) · F. Penault-Llorca (✉)
Department of Pathology and Molecular Pathology, Centre Jean Perrin, Clermont-Ferrand, France

UMR INSERM 1240, Universite Clermont Auvergne, Clermont-Ferrand, France
e-mail: myriam.kossai@clermont.unicancer.fr; frederique.penault-llorca@clermont.unicancer.fr

L. Deligdisch-Schor, A. Mareş Miceli (eds.), *Hormonal Pathology of the Uterus*, Advances in Experimental Medicine and Biology 1242,
https://doi.org/10.1007/978-3-030-38474-6_3

2 Leiomyoma

2.1 Definition, Epidemiology, Clinical Features

Uterine leiomyomas (ULs), often called fibroids or myomas, are benign smooth muscle tumors. They are the most common neoplasms in women, occurring in >70% of women worldwide [3, 4], but the true incidence is certainly underestimated. Histological studies on a series of uteri serially examined, resected for noncancerous conditions, showed that 56–77% of women had ULs [3, 5]. They mostly affect women during their reproductive age. Black women are particularly affected by ULs, with a higher prevalence and a two- to threefold incidence, occurring at a younger age than in Caucasian, Asian, and Hispanic women [4, 6, 7].

ULs occur in the uterine body (Fig. 1) but can develop in the cervix, uterine ligaments, and, rarely, the ovary and fallopian tube. A FIGO classification system has been established, based on tumor location (Fig. 2) [8]. They are well-demarcated lesions consisting of interlacing bundles of smooth muscle cells separated by substantial extracellular matrix (ECM) (Fig. 3). Histological examination defines the malignant potential of ULs by the assessment of nuclear grade and atypia, the count of mitoses, and the presence or absence of coagulative necrosis. Several subtypes have been described such as myxoid, epithelioid, cellular, and degenerated ULs (Fig. 4). Despite a low mitotic index, some subtypes present unusual growth patterns, commonly attributed to malignant lesions. These are diffuse leiomyomatosis, intravascular leiomyomatosis, benign metastasizing ULs, and disseminated peritoneal leiomyomatosis. For example, intravascular leiomyomatosis is a condition in which benign smooth muscle cells are present within the lumen of veins, which could spread to the heart without invading other tissues. Disseminated peritoneal

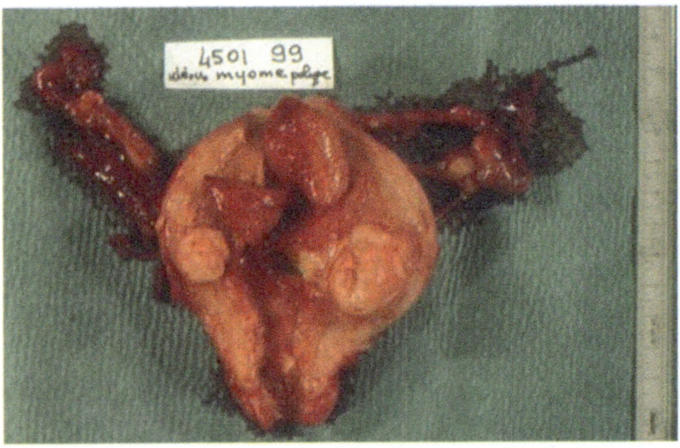

Fig. 1 Uterine leiomyomata (submucosal, intramural, and subserosal) and endometrial polyp

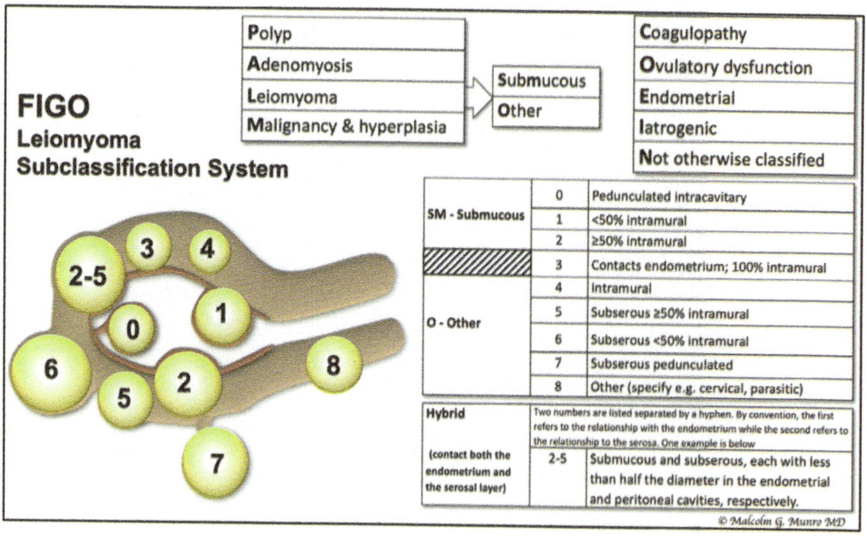

Fig. 2 The FIGO leiomyoma classification system. (From Munro et al. Int J Gynaecol Obstet. 2011)

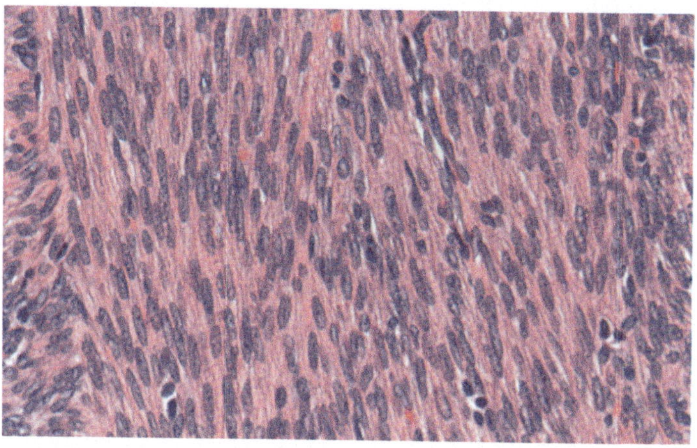

Fig. 3 Leiomyoma composed of spindle-shaped smooth muscle cells, with uniform, regular nuclei. H&E ×40

leiomyomatosis exhibits small nodular deposits of benign smooth muscle throughout the superficial subperitoneal tissues without tissue invasion.

Clinically, ULs are symptomatic in about one third of women over 30 years, rising to more than 40% in women over 40 years. They present with a variety of symptoms due mostly to their local mass effect. Heavy menstrual bleeding and pelvic pressure are the most common symptoms. Chronic pelvic pain, pressure upon adjacent organs resulting in incontinence, increased urinary frequency, and constipation

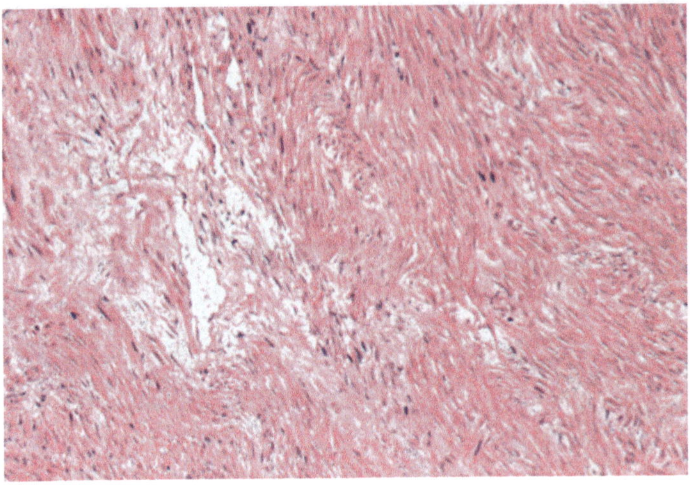

Fig. 4 Microscopic section of a leiomyoma with degenerative changes. H&E ×40

are commonly described. ULs can also cause problems related to pregnancy including infertility, early pregnancy loss, and later pregnancy complications [9]. The disease is more severe in black women compared to white women, with larger and more numerous tumors [7, 10].

The severity of symptoms depends on the number, size and location of the tumors in the uterus. ULs are often multiple and demonstrate a large heterogeneity even within the same woman, presenting several ULs showing different growth rates [3, 11].

As a consequence, ULs represent a major indication of hysterectomy and an important public health burden. As an example, the estimated annual healthcare-related costs of ULs range from 6 to 34 billion USD in the United States [12].

2.2 *Risk Factors and Etiopathogenesis*

A variety of risk factors that can overlap have been identified, from genetic and epigenetic factors to modifiable lifestyle factors [13, 14]. Increasing age until age of menopause and ethnicity (African ancestry) are the main factors. Family history of ULs, time since last birth, high blood pressure, obesity, soybean milk and food additive consumption, and vitamin C deficiency are other factors. Pregnancy (with a risk that decreases with an increasing number of pregnancies), oral contraceptive use, and smoking in women with a low BMI may lower the risk of ULs.

Other pathogenetic factors have also been reported such as growth factors, cytokines, chemokines, and extracellular matrix components. The role of steroid hormones remains decisive for the development and growth of ULs.

The ULs' etiology is unclear, certainly multifactorial; ULs derive from a proliferation of a single clone of smooth muscle cells [15, 16]. The myometrium and ULs contain multipotent somatic stem cells that represent a reservoir supporting growth and self-renewal [17]. Stem cells from ULs carry genetic mutations, whereas the myometrium does not, suggesting that a mutation as a first "hit" is required for the genesis of UL from a myometrial stem cell. Among genetic alterations, 12 trisomy, deletions in 7q, and mutations in genes encoding high mobility group AT-hook 2 (*HMGA2*) or mediator complex subunit 12 (*MED12*) have been reported [18–20]. The latter one is frequent, found in around 70% of ULs. In addition to sporadic alterations, ULs are a feature of hereditary leiomyomatosis and renal cancer syndrome (HLRCC) caused by heterozygous germline mutations in fumarate hydratase (*FH*) [21, 22].

ULs seem to develop in response to the menstrual cyclic steroid hormones. Estrogen and progesterone and their nuclear receptors (ER and PR, respectively) stimulate the genesis and growth of ULs. Messenger RNA and protein, estrogen and progesterone, and their receptor levels are higher in UL compared to those in normal myometrium [23–26]. Stem cells derived from ULs express low levels of estrogen and progesterone compared with UL cells or normal myometrial cells [27]. The growth of UL cells requires the surrounding myometrial cells with higher levels of steroid hormone receptors and their ligands, potentially mediated in a paracrine fashion [17]. Some studies showed that estrogen and progesterone activate several pathways such as the WNT/β-catenin pathway, leading to the stimulation of various transcription factors and downstream signaling, ultimately giving rise to the clonal proliferation of ULs [28–31]. Ovarian estrogen and estrogen induced locally by the aromatase activity are key regulators in UL cells. Aromatase inhibitors are efficient in reducing significantly UL size, showing that local aromatase activity is essential [32].

Progesterone is essential for maintenance and growth of ULs and, according to some studies, appears to be an even more important regulator than estrogen [33–36]. A study suggested that estrogen maintains PR levels and that progesterone, by interacting receptors, promotes UL growth [37]. Progesterone and progesterone receptors influence proliferation of ULs by regulating expression of growth factor signaling proteins such as epidermal growth factor (EGF) and signaling pathways. Progesterone receptors can directly bind to antiapoptotic BCL-2 promoter preventing apoptosis in UL cells [38–40]. The use of antiprogestins or selective progesterone receptor modulators in clinical trials provides yet the strongest evidence for the effect of progesterone on UL growth. Indeed, these treatments induced a decreased tumor size [35, 36, 41–44].

2.3 Treatment

Regarding UL treatment, there are no standard guidelines due to a lack of randomized controlled trials. Studies comparing treatment options are rare and follow-up investigation is often missing. The strategy depends on the presence or absence of symptoms and their nature (heavy menstrual bleeding, bulk symptoms, or both). For women with asymptomatic ULs, it is generally recommended to have follow-up evaluations. There is an exception for women with submucosal ULs who want future childbearing: hysteroscopic resection is indicated even if ULs are asymptomatic, according to some guidelines [45]. Although surgical interventions had historically been the mainstay in UL treatment, therapeutic options for symptomatic ULs also include medical and radiological procedures. However, a systematic review pointed out the lack of high-quality evidence supporting the effectiveness of most medical treatments [46].

2.3.1 Medical Treatment

For UL-related heavy bleeding, nonsteroid treatments include antifibrinolytics (tranexamic acid) and nonsteroidal anti-inflammatory drugs (NSAIDs) that have shown to be effective [47]. NSAIDs also reduce pain.

Contraceptive associate synthetic analogues of progesterone and estrogen are widely prescribed for the treatment of UL-related heavy menstrual bleeding.

Progesterone receptor agents are intended to reduce heavy menstrual bleeding by reducing endometrial hyperplasia associated with ULs. They include antiprogestins (mifepristone), selective progesterone receptor modulators (SPRMs, ulipristal acetate UPA), and levonorgestrel intrauterine device (LNG-IUD). UPA showed to be effective in decreasing ULs and uterine volume and improved symptoms such as pain and bleeding, most patients achieving amenorrhea [35, 36]. Because of specific pathological SPRM-related endometrial changes, an intermittent regimen is recommended [48]. These are also used for preoperative treatment of ULs. Hence, SPRMs are becoming the standard medical option for ULs with bulk symptoms. Studies assessing mifepristone showed a decrease in size of ULs and the total uterine volume at the completion of the period of active treatment. UL-related symptoms affecting the quality of life were also substantially improved [49, 50]. LNG-IUDs have been shown to reduce bleeding and to restore hemoglobin levels in women with ULs (except those that are submucosal) [51]. Mifepristone and LNG-IUDs have not been approved as therapy for ULs; further clinical trials to support their use are required [52].

Gonadotropin-releasing hormone (GnRH) agonists reduce the size of ULs and the overall uterine volume associated with a reduction of bleeding reported in some studies [53, 54]. Other symptoms such as pelvic pain and pressure, urinary frequency, and constipation were consistently ameliorated. Despite these positive effects, this treatment causes numerous side effects mimicking menopause, including vasomotor effects and bone mineral density loss, although some of these can be improved with hormonal "add-back" therapy using estrogens. Another problem resides in the fact that ULs recur following discontinuation of treatment. Hence, this drug is recommended for preoperative management for short periods [45, 55]. GnRH antagonists have similar effects with GnRH agonists with an immediate effect, avoiding the "flare-up" [56]. They reduce UL volume, but they do not improve bleeding and are not considered as an effective treatment for ULs.

Selective estrogen receptor modulator (SERM) raloxifene was assessed in randomized trial showing inconsistent results [57, 58]. Aromatase inhibitors showed to be effective in reducing ULs and uterine volume as well as symptoms [59]. Those agents are not currently supported for the treatments of ULs.

2.3.2 Interventional Procedures for ULs

Several studies randomized women to uterine artery embolization (UAE) procedure; this is a conservative approach and should be considered for women with symptomatic ULs. ULs and uterine volume decreased significantly as well as symptoms after UAE, regardless of the embolization agent or size of particles used to occlude the UL arteries [60]. The EMMY trial was a long-term follow-up report from the "Embolization for the Treatment of Symptomatic Uterine Fibroid Tumors" study and confirmed that ULs and uterine volume reductions persist up to 5 years after UAE; however, 28% (23/81) of women underwent subsequent hysterectomy [61].

Magnetic resonance-guided focused ultrasound (MRgFUS) is a noninvasive thermoablative technique, also effective in reducing UL size and symptoms, but remains experimental [62].

Laparoscopic radiofrequency UL ablation with intra-abdominal ultrasound guidance has been approved for the treatment of ULs with bulk symptoms [63, 64]. In addition, this procedure seems to result in less intraoperative blood loss and a shorter hospital stay, compared to myomectomy.

Myolysis using energy delivery systems based upon radiofrequency electricity or supercooled cryoprobes and laparoscopic ligations of the uterine arteries are other techniques used for women with UL-related bulk symptoms, but they need to be validated in clinical trials [45, 65].

2.3.3 Surgical Treatment

For women with intrauterine ULs (FIGO type 0, type 1, or type 2 up to 4 cm), myomectomy seems to be the best option for the treatment of UL-related bleeding [45]. It can be performed by hysteroscopy, laparoscopy or laparotomy. This technique removes ULs and preserves the uterus. However, patients must be informed that the symptoms may persist and ULs may recur, requiring further surgery. It is recommended in asymptomatic women who desire future fertility given its minimal morbidity.

Endometrial ablation is a minimally invasive procedure to be considered for women who wish to preserve fertility but as a second option after medical treatment since this technique increases the risk for extrauterine pregnancy [66].

Definitive hysterectomy is used following the failure of medical treatment in women with FIGO type 3 and higher ULs. It is recommended for women who do not intend to get pregnant. This method showed significant improvement in quality of life [45].

3 Adenomyosis

3.1 Definition, Epidemiology, Clinical Features

Adenomyosis is not considered a neoplasm but an endometrial disorder described as "the benign invasion of endometrium into the myometrium, producing a diffusely enlarged uterus which microscopically exhibits ectopic non-neoplastic, endometrial glands and stroma surrounded by the hypertrophic and hyperplastic myometrium" (Fig. 5) [67]. It was initially described by Carl von Rokitansky in 1860, before endometriosis, but the term was first used by Frankl in 1925. The endometrial-myometrial junction is irregular, the involvement of the superficial myometrium by endometrial mucosa occurring to varying degrees. Consequently "adenomyosis" is not well defined. The distance to which the endometrial tissue extends into the myometrium has been expressed as a number of microscopic fields from the junction. It has been commonly suggested that the diagnosis is based on a myometrial depth of ≥2.5 mm on one microscopic field at ten times magnification from the junction [68].

Adenomyosis occurs mostly in the late reproductive years, and its prevalence varies widely, with an average rate of 20–25% [69]. Recent studies showed that this condition is not particularly associated with other uterine disorders or neoplasms such as leiomyoma and prolapse [70].

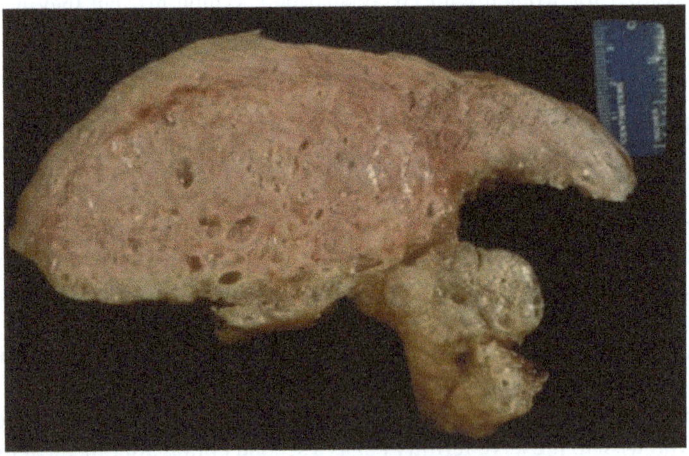

Fig. 5 Extensive adenomyosis in uterine cross section, with sponge-like appearance due to endometrial glands and their cystic hyperplasia (gross image)

Dysmenorrhea and dyspareunia are the most common symptoms, but the patient can be asymptomatic [71]. Pain, heavy periods, and infertility are other reported symptoms.

Until recently, adenomyosis could only be diagnosed by histology on hysterectomy. With the improvement of high-resolution ultrasound and the development of magnetic resonance imaging (MRI), the diagnosis of adenomyosis can now be relatively reliably made without a hysterectomy [72–74].

3.2 *Risk Factors, Etiopathogenesis*

Age, multiparity, and prior uterine surgery are the main risk factors involved in the etiology of adenomyosis [75]. The development of adenomyosis is influenced by steroids, but the pathogenetic mechanisms of adenomyosis remain unclear. Other factors which have been proposed to play a role in the etiopathogenesis of adenomyosis are inflammation, altered cell proliferation, and neoangiogenesis [76].

Regarding adenomyosis etiology, there are two main theories. Adenomyosis may develop from invagination of the endometrial basalis into the myometrium, through an altered or absent junctional zone [77]. This altered junctional zone presents week smooth muscle fibers that have loosened their tissue cohesion [78]. The invagination is due to activation of the tissue injury and repair (TIAR) mechanism, resulting in a local supraphysiological estrogen production in eutopic and ectopic endometrium in patients with adenomyosis. A higher level of estrogen was detected in menstrual blood but not in peripheral blood in women with this disease, corroborating these findings [79].

Gene polymorphisms such as catechol-O-methyltransferase (COMT), cytochrome P450–1B1 (CYP1B1), and COX-2 have been associated with the risk of developing adenomyosis [80, 81]. Progesterone and estrogen have antagonist effects. Some studies demonstrated that some epigenetic aberrations in progesterone receptor genes lead to a reduction or a loss of the progesterone receptor activity in women with adenomyosis [82, 83]. This hormonal deregulation indirectly increases estrogen-induced proliferation.

Postmenopausal women with breast cancer treated with tamoxifen have a higher rate of adenomyosis than those untreated [84]. By its estrogenic action, tamoxifen may promote the development of adenomyosis or its persistency in postmenopause [85]. Hence, hyperestrogenism promotes hyperperistalsis and increases local damage allowing the invagination of endometrial tissue into the myometrium [86–88].

The cycle of auto-traumatization worsens with each menstrual cycle, increasing the disruption of the muscular fibers and the “invasion” of the endometrium into the muscular uterine wall. Also, cesarean section, increased birth rates, and prior uterine surgery are risk factors for adenomyosis, supporting that tissue trauma plays a role in the pathogenesis of this disease [89–92].

The other hypothesis suggests that adenomyosis may originate from the differentiation of endometrial stem cells or de novo from metaplasia and displaced embryonic pluripotent Müllerian remnants [76, 93, 94]. This Müllerian metaplasia theory is supported by case reports of adenomyosis in hypoplastic myometrium of patients with Mayer-Rokitansky-Kuster-Hauser syndrome (absence of functional endometrium).

The other origin of metaplasia may lie in small populations of adult epithelial and stromal stem cells that have been reported in the uterus and are thought to differentiate [95]. These cells reside in the endometrial basalis within niches and have a clonogenic and progenitor activity responsible for the remarkable regenerative activity of the endometrium [93]. They may also have enhanced capacity to regenerate, leading to a dysregulation of endometrial stem cells, which could represent a mechanism for seeding ectopic endometrium into the myometrium. Endometrial stem cells may be deposited in the muscular wall due to retrograde menstruation containing endometrial fragments and then differentiate into endometrial tissue. Moreover, it has been suggested that adult stem cells could be activated by tissue injury promoting the disruption of stem cell niches in the junctional zone [93, 96]. Recently, Ibrahim et al. described a population of epithelial stem-like cells called "pale cells" in the basal endometrial glands [97]. These cells have motile properties and may represent the population that migrates actively into the myometrium, fostered by microscopic injury at the endometrial junctional zone.

3.3 *Treatment*

Several therapeutic options are available, from medical hormonal or nonhormonal treatments to nonconservative surgery, but to date there are no international guidelines. The choice depends on the woman's age, reproductive status, and clinical symptoms [98].

3.3.1 Steroidal Treatments

Adenomyosis is an estrogen-dependent condition that responds to hormonal treatment. The aim of medical treatment is to induce amenorrhea and inhibit ovulation, based on the theory that the responses of the eutopic and ectopic endometrium are substantially similar, leading to an improvement of the symptoms and a potential increase of fertility.

Oral estrogen-progestin contraceptives commonly used to treat adolescents cause decidualization and subsequent atrophy of the uterus, enabling long-term pain control and reducing menstruation.

GnRH agonists present antiproliferative and anti-inflammatory effects, reducing the uterine size and improving symptoms [99]. However, the use of GnRH agonists has hypoestrogenic side effects such as vasomotor syndrome, genital atrophy, mood instability, and reduced bone mineral density. To limit these side effects, an "add-back" therapy is recommended. Nonetheless, specific studies on this therapeutic regimen for the treatment of adenomyosis are lacking.

Progestins such as danazol, norethisterone acetate (NETA), and dienogest (DNG) have the same mechanism of actions as GnRHa and also induce a hypoestrogenism, having consequently the same effects. Unfortunately, there are limited data regarding the use of progestins in women with adenomyosis. Few retrospective and prospective studies showed a significant improvement in pelvic pain and bleeding [100–107].

Levonorgestrel-releasing intrauterine device (LNG-IUD) seems to be an effective long-term treatment. It leads to a reduction of menstruation and pain through a decidualization and an atrophy of the uterine wall and a reduction of uterine volume [108–110]. It acts directly on adenomyotic lesions by downregulating estrogen receptors [111]. Ozdegirmenci et al. compared the LNG-IUD with hysterectomy in adenomyosis patients, in a randomized controlled trial. After 6 months, the hemoglobin levels in both groups were similar and increased with LNG-IUD; this treatment has a superior effect on the quality of life compared to hysterectomy [112].

Selective estrogen receptor modulators (SERMs), selective progesterone receptor modulators (SPRMs), and aromatase inhibitors (AIs) are emerging drugs that show promising results [69], but supporting evidence for their clinical use is still necessary.

3.3.2 Nonsteroidal Medical Treatments

Nonsteroidal anti-inflammatory drugs (NSAIDs) are usually used to treat adenomyosis-related symptoms. Some systemic reviews showed that they are effective in treating menstrual pain and reducing menstrual blood loss [47, 113]; however, there are no studies investigating the use of NSAIDs in adenomyosis. Medical approaches can be ineffective and symptoms often relapse.

3.3.3 Interventional Procedures

Conservative treatment is required for women who wish to preserve their fertility. Uterine artery embolization (UAE) and MRI-guided focused ultrasound (MRgFUS) are conservative interventional procedures [114–116]. UAE has shown to be effective in the treatment of women with ULs and with both ULs and adenomyosis [117]. Several studies investigated the use of MRgFUS in women with symptomatic adenomyosis; this procedure appears to be effective and safe, but more clinical data is required [117].

3.3.4 Surgical Treatment

Minimally invasive surgical procedures are an alternative option when medical treatment is insufficient. Hysteroscopic excision of adenomyosis foci has been suggested before treatment for fertility. Results of studies on endometrial ablation of adenomyosis are conflicting [117]. This technique should not be used when foci of adenomyosis are deep, a major cause of treatment failure.

Surgical excision by laparoscopy of localized lesions sparing the uterus seemed to be safe. Hysterectomy is a definitive surgery and represents the gold standard treatment for women who have no desire for future fertility. Total hysterectomy should be favored over subtotal hysterectomy since there were few case reports of recurrence of the disease in the cervical stump or in the rectovaginal septum [118].

4 Endometrial Polyps

4.1 Definition, Epidemiology, Clinical Features

Endometrial polyps (EPs) are localized exophytic biphasic growths of endometrial glands and stroma with blood vessels protruding into the uterine cavity. They can arise at any age in about 13–17% of women but are more frequent shortly after menopause [119]. They can be single or multiple, measuring a few millimeters up to several centimeters, and can be sessile or pedunculated in shape (see Fig. 1). They can develop anywhere in the uterine cavity and can regress spontaneously [120]. EPs are in a large majority benign (Fig. 6), but atypical hyperplasia and adenocarcinoma, generally of the endometrioid type, may occur [121].

EPs are usually asymptomatic. They can be a cause of abnormal bleeding with no correlation with the polyp's size or growth rate [122].

4.2 Etiopathogenesis

Several hypotheses have been suggested regarding their pathogenesis. They may arise as monoclonal overgrowths of genetically altered stromal cells promoting proliferation of adjacent epithelial cells [123, 124]. Rearrangements in a high mobility group (HMG) family of transcription factors have been identified in EP [124–126]. It has been suggested that they can develop through a mechanism involving an aromatase-dependent focal hyperestrogenism [127, 128]. Ovarian hyperthecosis, a source of estrogen, may participate to the development of EPs in postmenopausal women [129]. EPs are related to hormonal imbalances; they can be functional show-

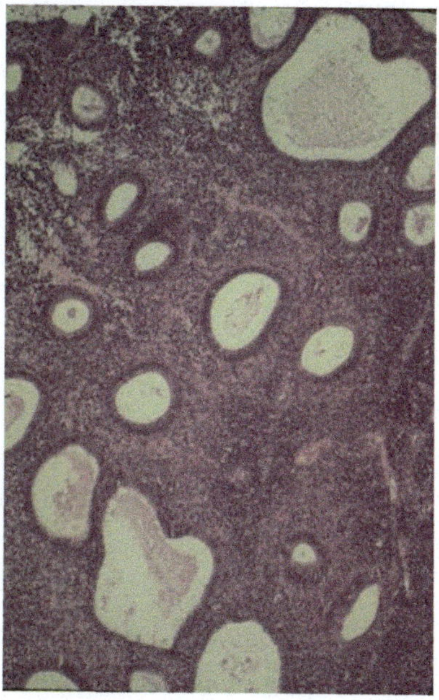

Fig. 6 Benign endometrial polyp with non-atypical glandular hyperplasia. H&E ×100

ing cycling changes in synchrony with those seen in the adjacent normal endometrium but more often are nonfunctional with no proliferative or secretory activity.

In recent years, the increasing age and the use of tamoxifen were the two most significant risk factors for the development of EPs (Fig. 7) [122]. Women on tamoxifen are more likely to present much larger, more fibrotic EPs, with mucinous metaplasia, and these EPs are more likely to contain hyperplasia or carcinoma [130].

Other risk factors have been reported in the pathogenesis of EPs, such as obesity, hypertension, and diabetes, but none of them is significant when women's age is taken into consideration [131].

EPs are associated with an increased risk of endometrial malignancy. Primary malignancy degeneration of a polyp occurs in 0.5–4.8% [132, 133]. EPs can also spontaneously regress over time, especially smaller ones (mean diameter 10.7 mm) compared to larger ones (mean diameters 15.1 mm), more frequently in premenopausal women [122].

4.3 Treatment

Current management of EPs depends on whether the patient is asymptomatic or not [134]. Some studies reported no correlation between polyp's growth rate, monitored by ultrasound scans, and symptoms. These findings suggest that routine ultrasound

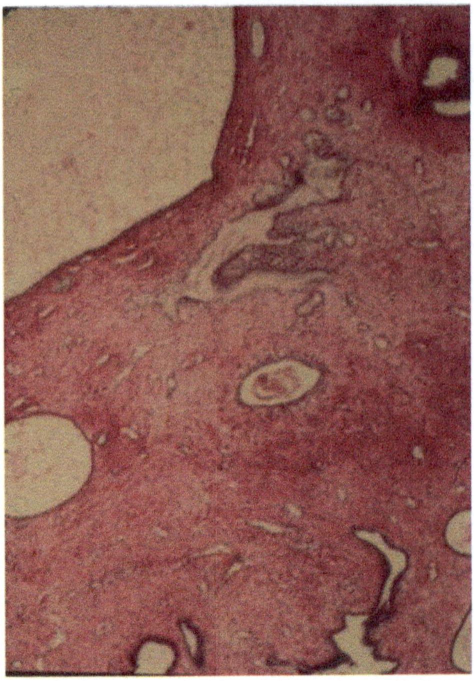

Fig. 7 Tamoxifen-treated patient with endometrial polyp showing cystic glands, mucinous metaplasia, and fibro-hyalinized stroma. H&E ×25

scans should not be used to predict the onset of symptoms and that patients with asymptomatic EP should report symptoms if they appear rather than having routine ultrasound scans [122].

EPs are generally removed by transcervical resection (TCRP) under hysteroscopy, a minimally invasive effective method, or by curettage or other sampling techniques such as pipelle [135]. When endometrial hyperplasia or adenocarcinoma is present on the specimen, the patient should be managed in the same way as if these premalignant and malignant lesions were found in a non-polypoid area.

Few studies have investigated the use of hormone therapy in the treatment of EPs after resection or the use of levonorgestrel-releasing intrauterine device, but significant clinical evidence supporting their use is needed [136, 137]. Currently, there is no recommended medical hormone therapy for the treatment of EPs.

5 Conclusions

Leiomyoma, adenomyosis, and endometrial polyps are common endometrial diseases. They share some common risk factors and symptoms such as heavy menstrual bleeding, pelvic pain, and a negative impact on women's quality of life. They also represent a significant health cost, particularly leiomyoma.

They seem to arise in a context of hormonal imbalances due to steroid hormones, estrogen and progesterone. A growing body of evidence suggests that those hormones and their receptors are key modulators in the genesis and the growth of those pathologic entities. Further studies are required to understand their involvement in the pathogenesis of those lesions and their link to other factors such as extracellular matrix components, growth factors, chemokines, cytokines, and tissue repair mechanisms. This will allow the identification of potential targets and co-targets for medical intervention.

Currently, medical therapies of leiomyoma and adenomyosis are focused on estrogen and progesterone receptors, showing significant results in decreasing symptoms and improving the quality of life of patients. Selective progesterone receptor modulators such as ulipristal acetate in the treatment of symptomatic leiomyoma demonstrated their efficacy in numerous studies and are currently available. Gonadotropin-releasing hormone agonists are used in preoperative treatment of leiomyoma. Steroidal treatment in adenomyosis showed consistent results, although, to date, there are no specific steroid therapy. For the treatment of endometrial polyp, transcervical resection remains the gold standard since these entities are easily resectable. In addition, most of them are nonfunctional, raising the possibility that hormonal treatment will not have any effect on their growth or their related symptoms.

References

1. Deneris A. PALM-COEIN nomenclature for abnormal uterine bleeding. J Midwifery Womens Health. 2016;61:376–9.
2. Munro MG. Uterine polyps, adenomyosis, leiomyomas, and endometrial receptivity. Fertil Steril. 2019;111:629–40.
3. Cramer SF, Patel A. The frequency of uterine leiomyomas. Am J Clin Pathol. 1990;94:435–8.
4. Baird DD, Dunson DB, Hill MC, Cousins D, Schectman JM. High cumulative incidence of uterine leiomyoma in black and white women: ultrasound evidence. Am J Obstet Gynecol. 2003;188:100–7.
5. Tiltman AJ. Smooth muscle neoplasms of the uterus. Curr Opin Obstet Gynecol. 1997;9:48–51.
6. Kjerulff KH, Langenberg P, Seidman JD, Stolley PD, Guzinski GM. Uterine leiomyomas. Racial differences in severity, symptoms and age at diagnosis. J Reprod Med. 1996;41:483–90.
7. Marshall LM, Spiegelman D, Barbieri RL, Goldman MB, Manson JE, Colditz GA, et al. Variation in the incidence of uterine leiomyoma among premenopausal women by age and race. Obstet Gynecol. 1997;90:967–73.
8. Munro MG, HOD C, Broder MS, Fraser IS, FIGO Working Group on Menstrual Disorders. FIGO classification system (PALM-COEIN) for causes of abnormal uterine bleeding in nongravid women of reproductive age. Int J Gynaecol Obstet. 2011;113:3–13.
9. Flake GP, Andersen J, Dixon D. Etiology and pathogenesis of uterine leiomyomas: a review. Environ Health Perspect. 2003;111:1037–54.
10. Huyck KL, Panhuysen CIM, Cuenco KT, Zhang J, Goldhammer H, Jones ES, et al. The impact of race as a risk factor for symptom severity and age at diagnosis of uterine leiomyomata among affected sisters. Am J Obstet Gynecol. 2008;198:168.e1–9.

11. Peddada SD, Laughlin SK, Miner K, Guyon J-P, Haneke K, Vahdat HL, et al. Growth of uterine leiomyomata among premenopausal black and white women. Proc Natl Acad Sci U S A. 2008;105:19887–92.
12. Cardozo ER, Clark AD, Banks NK, Henne MB, Stegmann BJ, Segars JH. The estimated annual cost of uterine leiomyomata in the United States. Am J Obstet Gynecol. 2012;206:211. e1–9.
13. Stewart EA, Cookson CL, Gandolfo RA, Schulze-Rath R. Epidemiology of uterine fibroids: a systematic review. BJOG Int J Obstet Gynaecol. 2017;124:1501–12.
14. Pavone D, Clemenza S, Sorbi F, Fambrini M, Petraglia F. Epidemiology and risk factors of uterine fibroids. Best Pract Res Clin Obstet Gynaecol. 2018;46:3–11.
15. Canevari RA, Pontes A, Rosa FE, Rainho CA, Rogatto SR. Independent clonal origin of multiple uterine leiomyomas that was determined by X chromosome inactivation and microsatellite analysis. Am J Obstet Gynecol. 2005;193:1395–403.
16. Zhang P, Zhang C, Hao J, Sung CJ, Quddus MR, Steinhoff MM, et al. Use of X-chromosome inactivation pattern to determine the clonal origins of uterine leiomyoma and leiomyosarcoma. Hum Pathol. 2006;37:1350–6.
17. Ono M, Qiang W, Serna VA, Yin P, Coon JS, Navarro A, et al. Role of stem cells in human uterine leiomyoma growth. PLoS One. 2012;7:e36935.
18. Mäkinen N, Mehine M, Tolvanen J, Kaasinen E, Li Y, Lehtonen HJ, et al. MED12, the mediator complex subunit 12 gene, is mutated at high frequency in uterine leiomyomas. Science. 2011;334:252–5.
19. Markowski DN, Bartnitzke S, Löning T, Drieschner N, Helmke BM, Bullerdiek J. MED12 mutations in uterine fibroids—their relationship to cytogenetic subgroups. Int J Cancer. 2012;131:1528–36.
20. Kämpjärvi K, Mäkinen N, Mehine M, Välipakka S, Uimari O, Pitkänen E, et al. MED12 mutations and FH inactivation are mutually exclusive in uterine leiomyomas. Br J Cancer. 2016;114:1405–11.
21. Launonen V, Vierimaa O, Kiuru M, Isola J, Roth S, Pukkala E, et al. Inherited susceptibility to uterine leiomyomas and renal cell cancer. Proc Natl Acad Sci U S A. 2001;98:3387–92.
22. Tomlinson IPM, Alam NA, Rowan AJ, Barclay E, Jaeger EEM, Kelsell D, et al. Germline mutations in FH predispose to dominantly inherited uterine fibroids, skin leiomyomata and papillary renal cell cancer. Nat Genet. 2002;30:406–10.
23. Kovács KA, Oszter A, Göcze PM, Környei JL, Szabó I. Comparative analysis of cyclin D1 and oestrogen receptor (alpha and beta) levels in human leiomyoma and adjacent myometrium. Mol Hum Reprod. 2001;7:1085–91.
24. Ying Z, Weiyuan Z. Dual actions of progesterone on uterine leiomyoma correlate with the ratio of progesterone receptor A:B. Gynecol Endocrinol. 2009;25:520–3.
25. Viville B, Charnock-Jones DS, Sharkey AM, Wetzka B, Smith SK. Distribution of the A and B forms of the progesterone receptor messenger ribonucleic acid and protein in uterine leiomyomata and adjacent myometrium. Hum Reprod. 1997;12:815–22.
26. Benassayag C, Leroy MJ, Rigourd V, Robert B, Honoré JC, Mignot TM, et al. Estrogen receptors (ERalpha/ERbeta) in normal and pathological growth of the human myometrium: pregnancy and leiomyoma. Am J Phys. 1999;276:E1112–8.
27. Bulun SE. Uterine fibroids. N Engl J Med. 2013;369:1344–55.
28. Tai C-T, Lin W-C, Chang W-C, Chiu T-H, Chen GTC. Classical cadherin and catenin expression in normal myometrial tissues and uterine leiomyomas. Mol Reprod Dev. 2003;64:172–8.
29. Tanwar PS, Lee H-J, Zhang L, Zukerberg LR, Taketo MM, Rueda BR, et al. Constitutive activation of beta-catenin in uterine stroma and smooth muscle leads to the development of mesenchymal tumors in mice. Biol Reprod. 2009;81:545–52.
30. Mosimann C, Hausmann G, Basler K. Beta-catenin hits chromatin: regulation of Wnt target gene activation. Nat Rev Mol Cell Biol. 2009;10:276–86.
31. Arici A, Sozen I. Transforming growth factor-beta3 is expressed at high levels in leiomyoma where it stimulates fibronectin expression and cell proliferation. Fertil Steril. 2000;73:1006–11.

32. Parsanezhad ME, Azmoon M, Alborzi S, Rajaeefard A, Zarei A, Kazerooni T, et al. A randomized, controlled clinical trial comparing the effects of aromatase inhibitor (letrozole) and gonadotropin-releasing hormone agonist (triptorelin) on uterine leiomyoma volume and hormonal status. Fertil Steril. 2010;93:192–8.
33. Kastner P, Krust A, Turcotte B, Stropp U, Tora L, Gronemeyer H, et al. Two distinct estrogen-regulated promoters generate transcripts encoding the two functionally different human progesterone receptor forms A and B. EMBO J. 1990;9:1603–14.
34. Kim JJ, Sefton EC. The role of progesterone signaling in the pathogenesis of uterine leiomyoma. Mol Cell Endocrinol. 2012;358:223–31.
35. Donnez J, Tomaszewski J, Vázquez F, Bouchard P, Lemieszczuk B, Baró F, et al. Ulipristal acetate versus leuprolide acetate for uterine fibroids. N Engl J Med. 2012;366:421–32.
36. Donnez J, Tatarchuk TF, Bouchard P, Puscasiu L, Zakharenko NF, Ivanova T, et al. Ulipristal acetate versus placebo for fibroid treatment before surgery. N Engl J Med. 2012;366:409–20.
37. Ishikawa H, Ishi K, Serna VA, Kakazu R, Bulun SE, Kurita T. Progesterone is essential for maintenance and growth of uterine leiomyoma. Endocrinology. 2010;151:2433–42.
38. Ohara N, Morikawa A, Chen W, Wang J, DeManno DA, Chwalisz K, et al. Comparative effects of SPRM asoprisnil (J867) on proliferation, apoptosis, and the expression of growth factors in cultured uterine leiomyoma cells and normal myometrial cells. Reprod Sci. 2007;14:20–7.
39. Chen W, Ohara N, Wang J, Xu Q, Liu J, Morikawa A, et al. A novel selective progesterone receptor modulator asoprisnil (J867) inhibits proliferation and induces apoptosis in cultured human uterine leiomyoma cells in the absence of comparable effects on myometrial cells. J Clin Endocrinol Metab. 2006;91:1296–304.
40. Hoekstra AV, Sefton EC, Berry E, Lu Z, Hardt J, Marsh E, et al. Progestins activate the AKT pathway in leiomyoma cells and promote survival. J Clin Endocrinol Metab. 2009;94:1768–74.
41. Bagaria M, Suneja A, Vaid NB, Guleria K, Mishra K. Low-dose mifepristone in treatment of uterine leiomyoma: a randomised double-blind placebo-controlled clinical trial. Aust N Z J Obstet Gynaecol. 2009;49:77–83.
42. Williams ARW, Critchley HOD, Osei J, Ingamells S, Cameron IT, Han C, et al. The effects of the selective progesterone receptor modulator asoprisnil on the morphology of uterine tissues after 3 months treatment in patients with symptomatic uterine leiomyomata. Hum Reprod. 2007;22:1696–704.
43. Engman M, Granberg S, Williams ARW, Meng CX, Lalitkumar PGL, Gemzell-Danielsson K. Mifepristone for treatment of uterine leiomyoma. A prospective randomized placebo controlled trial. Hum Reprod. 2009;24:1870–9.
44. Eisinger SH, Meldrum S, Fiscella K, le Roux HD, Guzick DS. Low-dose mifepristone for uterine leiomyomata. Obstet Gynecol. 2003;101:243–50.
45. Marret H, Fritel X, Ouldamer L, Bendifallah S, Brun J-L, De Jesus I, et al. Therapeutic management of uterine fibroid tumors: updated French guidelines. Eur J Obstet Gynecol Reprod Biol. 2012;165:156–64.
46. Gliklich RE, Leavy MB, Velentgas P, Campion DM, Mohr P, Sabharwal R, et al. Identification of Future Research Needs in the Comparative Management of Uterine Fibroid Disease. Effective Health Care Program. https://effectivehealthcare.ahrq.gov/topics/uterine-fibroids-2010/research
47. Lethaby A, Duckitt K, Farquhar C. Non-steroidal anti-inflammatory drugs for heavy menstrual bleeding. Cochrane Database Syst Rev. 2013;(1):CD000400.
48. Mutter GL, Bergeron C, Deligdisch L, Ferenczy A, Glant M, Merino M, et al. The spectrum of endometrial pathology induced by progesterone receptor modulators. Mod Pathol. 2008;21:591–8.
49. Tristan M, Orozco LJ, Steed A, Ramírez-Morera A, Stone P. Mifepristone for uterine fibroids. Cochrane Database Syst Rev. 2012;(8):CD007687.
50. Shen Q, Hua Y, Jiang W, Zhang W, Chen M, Zhu X. Effects of mifepristone on uterine leiomyoma in premenopausal women: a meta-analysis. Fertil Steril. 2013;100:1722–6.e1–10.

51. Sangkomkamhang US, Lumbiganon P, Laopaiboon M, Mol BWJ. Progestogens or progestogen-releasing intrauterine systems for uterine fibroids. Cochrane Database Syst Rev. 2013;(2):CD008994.
52. Steinauer J, Pritts EA, Jackson R, Jacoby AF. Systematic review of mifepristone for the treatment of uterine leiomyomata. Obstet Gynecol. 2004;103:1331–6.
53. Muzii L, Boni T, Bellati F, Marana R, Ruggiero A, Zullo MA, et al. GnRH analogue treatment before hysteroscopic resection of submucous myomas: a prospective, randomized, multicenter study. Fertil Steril. 2010;94:1496–9.
54. Lethaby AE, Vollenhoven BJ. An evidence-based approach to hormonal therapies for premenopausal women with fibroids. Best Pract Res Clin Obstet Gynaecol. 2008;22:307–31.
55. Laughlin-Tommaso SK, Stewart EA. Moving toward individualized medicine for uterine leiomyomas. Obstet Gynecol. 2018;132:961–71.
56. Flierman PA, Oberyé JJL, van der Hulst VPM, de Blok S. Rapid reduction of leiomyoma volume during treatment with the GnRH antagonist ganirelix. BJOG Int J Obstet Gynaecol. 2005;112:638–42.
57. Palomba S, Orio F, Morelli M, Russo T, Pellicano M, Zupi E, et al. Raloxifene administration in premenopausal women with uterine leiomyomas: a pilot study. J Clin Endocrinol Metab. 2002;87:3603–8.
58. Palomba S, Russo T, Orio F, Tauchmanovà L, Zupi E, Panici PLB, et al. Effectiveness of combined GnRH analogue plus raloxifene administration in the treatment of uterine leiomyomas: a prospective, randomized, single-blind, placebo-controlled clinical trial. Hum Reprod. 2002;17:3213–9.
59. Hilário SG, Bozzini N, Borsari R, Baracat EC. Action of aromatase inhibitor for treatment of uterine leiomyoma in perimenopausal patients. Fertil Steril. 2009;91:240–3.
60. Hartmann KE, Fonnesbeck C, Surawicz T, Krishnaswami S, Andrews JC, Wilson JE, et al. Management of Uterine Fibroids [Internet]. Rockville (MD): Agency for Healthcare Research and Quality (US); http://www.ncbi.nlm.nih.gov/books/NBK537742/
61. Hehenkamp WJK, Volkers NA, Donderwinkel PFJ, de Blok S, Birnie E, Ankum WM, et al. Uterine artery embolization versus hysterectomy in the treatment of symptomatic uterine fibroids (EMMY trial): peri- and postprocedural results from a randomized controlled trial. Am J Obstet Gynecol. 2005;193:1618–29.
62. Peregrino PFM, de Lorenzo Messina M, dos Santos Simões R, Soares-Júnior JM, Baracat EC. Review of magnetic resonance-guided focused ultrasound in the treatment of uterine fibroids. Clinics. 2017;72:637–41.
63. Brucker SY, Hahn M, Kraemer D, Taran FA, Isaacson KB, Krämer B. Laparoscopic radiofrequency volumetric thermal ablation of fibroids versus laparoscopic myomectomy. Int J Gynaecol Obstet. 2014;125:261–5.
64. Lee BB, Yu SP. Radiofrequency ablation of uterine fibroids: a review. Curr Obstet Gynecol Rep. 2016;5:318–24.
65. Krämer B, Hahn M, Taran F-A, Kraemer D, Isaacson KB, Brucker SY. Interim analysis of a randomized controlled trial comparing laparoscopic radiofrequency volumetric thermal ablation of uterine fibroids with laparoscopic myomectomy. Int J Gynaecol Obstet. 2016;133:206–11.
66. Stewart EA, Laughlin-Tommaso SK, Catherino WH, Lalitkumar S, Gupta D, Vollenhoven B. Uterine fibroids. Nat Rev Dis Primer. 2016;2:16043.
67. Bird CC, McElin TW, Manalo-Estrella P. The elusive adenomyosis of the uterus—revisited. Am J Obstet Gynecol. 1972;112:583–93.
68. Seidman JD, Kjerulff KH. Pathologic findings from the Maryland Women's Health Study: practice patterns in the diagnosis of adenomyosis. Int J Gynecol Pathol. 1996;15:217–21.
69. Pontis A, D'Alterio MN, Pirarba S, de Angelis C, Tinelli R, Angioni S. Adenomyosis: a systematic review of medical treatment. Gynecol Endocrinol. 2016;32:696–700.
70. Hever A, Roth RB, Hevezi PA, Lee J, Willhite D, White EC, et al. Molecular characterization of human adenomyosis. Mol Hum Reprod. 2006;12:737–48.

71. Farquhar C, Brosens I. Medical and surgical management of adenomyosis. Best Pract Res Clin Obstet Gynaecol. 2006;20:603–16.
72. Bazot M, Daraï E. Role of transvaginal sonography and magnetic resonance imaging in the diagnosis of uterine adenomyosis. Fertil Steril. 2018;109:389–97.
73. Grimbizis GF, Mikos T, Tarlatzis B. Uterus-sparing operative treatment for adenomyosis. Fertil Steril. 2014;101:472–87.
74. Kishi Y, Suginami H, Kuramori R, Yabuta M, Suginami R, Taniguchi F. Four subtypes of adenomyosis assessed by magnetic resonance imaging and their specification. Am J Obstet Gynecol. 2012;207:114.e1–7.
75. Taran FA, Stewart EA, Brucker S. Adenomyosis: epidemiology, risk factors, clinical phenotype and surgical and interventional alternatives to hysterectomy. Geburtshilfe Frauenheilkd. 2013;73:924–31.
76. Vannuccini S, Tosti C, Carmona F, Huang SJ, Chapron C, Guo S-W, et al. Pathogenesis of adenomyosis: an update on molecular mechanisms. Reprod Biomed Online. 2017;35:592–601.
77. Bergeron C, Amant F, Ferenczy A. Pathology and physiopathology of adenomyosis. Best Pract Res Clin Obstet Gynaecol. 2006;20:511–21.
78. Brosens JJ, de Souza NM, Barker FG. Uterine junctional zone: function and disease. Lancet Lond Engl. 1995;346:558–60.
79. Takahashi K, Nagata H, Kitao M. Clinical usefulness of determination of estradiol level in the menstrual blood for patients with endometriosis. Nihon Sanka Fujinka Gakkai Zasshi. 1989;41:1849–50.
80. Tong X, Li Z, Wu Y, Fu X, Zhang Y, Fan H. COMT 158G/A and CYP1B1 432C/G polymorphisms increase the risk of endometriosis and adenomyosis: a meta-analysis. Eur J Obstet Gynecol Reprod Biol. 2014;179:17–21.
81. Wang Y, Qu Y, Song W. Genetic variation in COX-2 -1195 and the risk of endometriosis and adenomyosis. Clin Exp Obstet Gynecol. 2015;42:168–72.
82. Nie J, Liu X, Guo S-W. Promoter hypermethylation of progesterone receptor isoform B (PR-B) in adenomyosis and its rectification by a histone deacetylase inhibitor and a demethylation agent. Reprod Sci. 2010;17:995–1005.
83. Mehasseb MK, Panchal R, Taylor AH, Brown L, Bell SC, Habiba M. Estrogen and progesterone receptor isoform distribution through the menstrual cycle in uteri with and without adenomyosis. Fertil Steril. 2011;95:2228–35, 2235.e1.
84. Cohen I, Shapira J, Beyth Y, Bernheim J, Tepper R, Cordoba M, et al. Estrogen and progesterone receptors of adenomyosis in postmenopausal breast cancer patients treated with tamoxifen. Gynecol Obstet Investig. 1998;45:126–31.
85. McCluggage WG, Desai V, Manek S. Tamoxifen-associated postmenopausal adenomyosis exhibits stromal fibrosis, glandular dilatation and epithelial metaplasias. Histopathology. 2000;37:340–6.
86. Leyendecker G, Wildt L. A new concept of endometriosis and adenomyosis: tissue injury and repair (TIAR). Horm Mol Biol Clin Investig. 2011;5:125–42.
87. García-Solares J, Donnez J, Donnez O, Dolmans M-M. Pathogenesis of uterine adenomyosis: invagination or metaplasia? Fertil Steril. 2018;109:371–9.
88. Leyendecker G, Wildt L, Mall G. The pathophysiology of endometriosis and adenomyosis: tissue injury and repair. Arch Gynecol Obstet. 2009;280:529–38.
89. Riggs JC, Lim EK, Liang D, Bullwinkel R. Cesarean section as a risk factor for the development of adenomyosis uteri. J Reprod Med. 2014;59:20–4.
90. Parazzini F, Vercellini P, Panazza S, Chatenoud L, Oldani S, Crosignani PG. Risk factors for adenomyosis. Hum Reprod. 1997;12:1275–9.
91. Templeman C, Marshall SF, Ursin G, Horn-Ross PL, Clarke CA, Allen M, et al. Adenomyosis and endometriosis in the California Teachers Study. Fertil Steril. 2008;90:415–24.
92. Taran FA, Weaver AL, Coddington CC, Stewart EA. Understanding adenomyosis: a case control study. Fertil Steril. 2010;94:1223–8.
93. Gargett CE. Uterine stem cells: what is the evidence? Hum Reprod Update. 2007;13:87–101.

94. Ferenczy A. Pathophysiology of adenomyosis. Hum Reprod Update. 1998;4:312–22.
95. Chan RWS, Schwab KE, Gargett CE. Clonogenicity of human endometrial epithelial and stromal cells. Biol Reprod. 2004;70:1738–50.
96. Gargett CE, Schwab KE, Deane JA. Endometrial stem/progenitor cells: the first 10 years. Hum Reprod Update. 2016;22:137–63.
97. Ibrahim MG, Chiantera V, Frangini S, Younes S, Köhler C, Taube ET, et al. Ultramicrotrauma in the endometrial-myometrial junctional zone and pale cell migration in adenomyosis. Fertil Steril. 2015;104:1475–1483.e3.
98. Vannuccini S, Petraglia F. Recent advances in understanding and managing adenomyosis. F1000Research 2019, 8(F1000 Faculty Rev):283 Last updated: 17 JUL 2019. https://f1000research.com/articles/8-28
99. Angioni S, Pontis A, Dessole M, Surico D, De Cicco Nardone C, Melis I. Pain control and quality of life after laparoscopic en-block resection of deep infiltrating endometriosis (DIE) vs. incomplete surgical treatment with or without GnRHa administration after surgery. Arch Gynecol Obstet. 2015;291:363–70.
100. Fawzy M, Mesbah Y. Comparison of dienogest versus triptorelin acetate in premenopausal women with adenomyosis: a prospective clinical trial. Arch Gynecol Obstet. 2015;292:1267–71.
101. Igarashi M. A new therapy for pelvic endometriosis and uterine adenomyosis: local effect of vaginal and intrauterine danazol application. Asia Oceania J Obstet Gynaecol. 1990;16:1–12.
102. Luisi S, Razzi S, Lazzeri L, Bocchi C, Severi FM, Petraglia F. Efficacy of vaginal danazol treatment in women with menorrhagia during fertile age. Fertil Steril. 2009;92:1351–4.
103. Muneyyirci-Delale O, Chandrareddy A, Mankame S, Osei-Tutu N, von Gizycki H. Norethindrone acetate in the medical management of adenomyosis. Pharmaceuticals. 2012;5:1120–7.
104. Sasagawa S, Shimizu Y, Kami H, Takeuchi T, Mita S, Imada K, et al. Dienogest is a selective progesterone receptor agonist in transactivation analysis with potent oral endometrial activity due to its efficient pharmacokinetic profile. Steroids. 2008;73:222–31.
105. Takebayashi T, Fujino Y, Umesaki N, Ogita S. Danazol suspension injected into the uterine cervix of patients with adenomyosis and myoma. Preliminary study. Gynecol Obstet Invest. 1995;39:207–11.
106. Tosti C, Vannuccini S, Troìa L, Luisi S, Centini G, Lazzeri L, et al. Long-term vaginal danazol treatment in fertile age women with adenomyosis. J Endometr Pelvic Pain Disord. 2017;9:39–43.
107. Zhang X, Yuan H, Deng L, Hu F, Ma J, Lin J. Evaluation of the efficacy of a danazol-loaded intrauterine contraceptive device on adenomyosis in an ICR mouse model. Hum Reprod. 2008;23:2024–30.
108. Fedele L, Bianchi S, Raffaelli R, Portuese A, Dorta M. Treatment of adenomyosis-associated menorrhagia with a levonorgestrel-releasing intrauterine device. Fertil Steril. 1997;68:426–9.
109. Fraser IS. Non-contraceptive health benefits of intrauterine hormonal systems. Contraception. 2010;82:396–403.
110. Sabbioni L, Petraglia F, Luisi S. Non-contraceptive benefits of intrauterine levonorgestrel administration: why not? Gynecol Endocrinol. 2017;33:822–9.
111. Fong YF, Singh K. Medical treatment of a grossly enlarged adenomyotic uterus with the levonorgestrel-releasing intrauterine system. Contraception. 1999;60:173–5.
112. Ozdegirmenci O, Kayikcioglu F, Akgul MA, Kaplan M, Karcaaltincaba M, Haberal A, et al. Comparison of levonorgestrel intrauterine system versus hysterectomy on efficacy and quality of life in patients with adenomyosis. Fertil Steril. 2011;95:497–502.
113. Marjoribanks J, Proctor M, Farquhar C, Derks RS. Nonsteroidal anti-inflammatory drugs for dysmenorrhoea. Cochrane Database Syst Rev. 2010;(1):CD001751.
114. Brosens I, Gordts S, Habiba M, Benagiano G. Uterine cystic adenomyosis: a disease of younger women. J Pediatr Adolesc Gynecol. 2015;28:420–6.

115. Gordts S, Campo R, Brosens I. Hysteroscopic diagnosis and excision of myometrial cystic adenomyosis. Gynecol Surg. 2014;11:273–8.
116. Kriplani A, Mahey R, Agarwal N, Bhatla N, Yadav R, Singh MK. Laparoscopic management of juvenile cystic adenomyoma: four cases. J Minim Invasive Gynecol. 2011;18:343–8.
117. Dueholm M. Uterine adenomyosis and infertility, review of reproductive outcome after in vitro fertilization and surgery. Acta Obstet Gynecol Scand. 2017;96:715–26.
118. Pepas L, Deguara C, Davis C. Update on the surgical management of adenomyosis. Curr Opin Obstet Gynecol. 2012;24:259–64.
119. Kim K-R, Peng R, Ro JY, Robboy SJ. A diagnostically useful histopathologic feature of endometrial polyp: the long axis of endometrial glands arranged parallel to surface epithelium. Am J Surg Pathol. 2004;28:1057–62.
120. de Rijk SR, Steenbergen ME, Nieboer TE, Coppus SF. Atypical endometrial polyps and concurrent endometrial cancer: a systematic review. Obstet Gynecol. 2016;128:519–25.
121. Kelly P, Dobbs SP, McCluggage WG. Endometrial hyperplasia involving endometrial polyps: report of a series and discussion of the significance in an endometrial biopsy specimen. BJOG Int J Obstet Gynaecol. 2007;114:944–50.
122. Wong M, Crnobrnja B, Liberale V, Dharmarajah K, Widschwendter M, Jurkovic D. The natural history of endometrial polyps. Hum Reprod. 2017;32:340–5.
123. Fletcher JA, Pinkus JL, Lage JM, Morton CC, Pinkus GS. Clonal 6p21 rearrangement is restricted to the mesenchymal component of an endometrial polyp. Genes Chromosomes Cancer. 1992;5:260–3.
124. Dal Cin P, Vanni R, Marras S, Moerman P, Kools P, Andria M, et al. Four cytogenetic subgroups can be identified in endometrial polyps. Cancer Res. 1995;55:1565–8.
125. Tallini G, Vanni R, Manfioletti G, Kazmierczak B, Faa G, Pauwels P, et al. HMGI-C and HMGI(Y) immunoreactivity correlates with cytogenetic abnormalities in lipomas, pulmonary chondroid hamartomas, endometrial polyps, and uterine leiomyomas and is compatible with rearrangement of the HMGI-C and HMGI(Y) genes. Lab Investig J Tech Methods Pathol. 2000;80:359–69.
126. Dal Cin P, Timmerman D, Van den Berghe I, Wanschura S, Kazmierczak B, Vergote I, et al. Genomic changes in endometrial polyps associated with tamoxifen show no evidence for its action as an external carcinogen. Cancer Res. 1998;58:2278–81.
127. Maia H, Pimentel K, Silva TMC, Freitas LAR, Zausner B, Athayde C, et al. Aromatase and cyclooxygenase-2 expression in endometrial polyps during the menstrual cycle. Gynecol Endocrinol. 2006;22:219–24.
128. Pal L, Niklaus AL, Kim M, Pollack S, Santoro N. Heterogeneity in endometrial expression of aromatase in polyp-bearing uteri. Hum Reprod. 2008;23:80–4.
129. Zhang C, Sung CJ, Quddus MR, Simon RA, Jazaerly T, Lawrence WD. Association of ovarian hyperthecosis with endometrial polyp, endometrial hyperplasia, and endometrioid adenocarcinoma in postmenopausal women: a clinicopathological study of 238 cases. Hum Pathol. 2017;59:120–4.
130. Berlière M, Radikov G, Galant C, Piette P, Marbaix E, Donnez J. Identification of women at high risk of developing endometrial cancer on tamoxifen. Eur J Cancer. 2000;36(Suppl 4):S35–6.
131. Nappi L, Indraccolo U, Di Spiezio Sardo A, Gentile G, Palombino K, Castaldi MA, et al. Are diabetes, hypertension, and obesity independent risk factors for endometrial polyps? J Minim Invasive Gynecol. 2009;16:157–62.
132. Lee SC, Kaunitz AM, Sanchez-Ramos L, Rhatigan RM. The oncogenic potential of endometrial polyps: a systematic review and meta-analysis. Obstet Gynecol. 2010;116:1197–205.
133. Goldstein SR, Monteagudo A, Popiolek D, Mayberry P, Timor-Tritsch I. Evaluation of endometrial polyps. Am J Obstet Gynecol. 2002;186:669–74.

134. Salim S, Won H, Nesbitt-Hawes E, Campbell N, Abbott J. Diagnosis and management of endometrial polyps: a critical review of the literature. J Minim Invasive Gynecol. 2011;18:569–81.
135. Savelli L, De Iaco P, Santini D, Rosati F, Ghi T, Pignotti E, et al. Histopathologic features and risk factors for benignity, hyperplasia, and cancer in endometrial polyps. Am J Obstet Gynecol. 2003;188:927–31.
136. Li F, Wei S, Yang S, Liu Z, Nan F. Post hysteroscopic progesterone hormone therapy in the treatment of endometrial polyps. Pak J Med Sci. 2018;34:1267–71.
137. Arnes M, Hvingel B, Orbo A. Levonorgestrel-impregnated intrauterine device reduces occurrence of hyperplastic polyps: a population-based follow-up cohort study. Anticancer Res. 2014;34:2319–24.

Endometrial Carcinoma and its Precursors

Pouya Javadian and Farr Nezhat

1 Introduction

Endometrial cancer affects mainly postmenopausal women. The average age of women diagnosed with endometrial cancer is 62; it is uncommon in women under the age of 45. This cancer is slightly more common in white women, but the incidence rate increase was higher in blacks, likely because black women in the United States appear to undergo hysterectomy at higher rates than white women. However, mortality was almost twofold higher in blacks than in whites (7.1 vs. 3.9 per 100,000 patients), possibly due to a higher incidence of aggressive cancer subtypes, as well as issues of access to and quality of healthcare services [1].

Obesity (BMI > 30), nulliparity, and late menopause or exogenous estrogen without adequate opposition by a progestin are known risk factors for endometrial carcinoma. Patients who received selective estrogen receptor modulator (SERM) tamoxifen and raloxifene and, more recently, aromatase inhibitors are also at increased risk of developing endometrial carcinoma. Another condition leading to long-term estrogen stimulation of the endometrium is the polycystic ovary

P. Javadian
Robert Wood Johnson Barnabas Health Newark Beth Israel Medical Center, Newark, NJ, USA

F. Nezhat (✉)
Nezhat Surgery for Gynecology/Oncology, New York, NY, USA

Weill Cornell Medical College of Cornell University, New York, NY, USA

Stony Brook University School of Medicine, Stony Brook, NY, USA

Department of Minimally Invasive Gynecologic Surgery and Robotics, NYU Winthrop University Hospital, Mineola, NY, USA
e-mail: farr@farrnezhatmd.com

L. Deligdisch-Schor, A. Mareş Miceli (eds.), *Hormonal Pathology of the Uterus*, Advances in Experimental Medicine and Biology 1242,
https://doi.org/10.1007/978-3-030-38474-6_4

syndrome. In addition, women with Lynch syndrome (hereditary nonpolyposis colon cancer) are at a markedly increased risk of endometrial cancer [2].

In the early 1980s, Bokhman suggested that there are two pathogenic types of endometrial cancer, type I and type II. While the majority of tumors are type I endometrioid carcinomas (EC), developing from and associated with atypical glandular hyperplasia, and related to prolonged unopposed estrogen effect, type II endometrial carcinomas may develop from atrophic endometrium. Occasionally an early stage of type II EC is detected, endometrial intraepithelial carcinoma (EIC)—as opposed to endometrial intraepithelial neoplasm (EIN), a precursor of type I EC. Type II EC are more aggressive tumors, often detected in late stages and not necessarily related to estrogen effect, as they are seen in multiparous, nonobese, mostly older patients. Their etiology is less clear, with possible genetic and environmental factors involved. Recent studies of human mammary tumor virus (HMTV) have identified viral envelope particles in the endometrial cancer epithelial cells in 23% of the examined cases, suggesting a possible cofactor via downstream effect [3].

Endometrial hyperplasia is characterized by a proliferation of endometrial glands resulting in a greater gland-to-stroma ratio (>50%) than observed in normal proliferative endometrium. The proliferating glands vary in size and shape, and cells may have cytologic atypia. Atypical hyperplasia results from increased estrogenic stimulation of the endometrium and is a precursor of endometrioid endometrial cancer. Unopposed estrogen stimulation yields a continuous spectrum of changes, ranging from proliferative endometrium to endometrial hyperplasia. Endometrial cancer is defined by the ability to invade local tissue and metastasize. Histopathologic classification of endometrial lesions provides a stratification of risk for progression to cancer by defined endometrial changes.

Type I endometrial carcinoma arises in women with obesity, hyperlipidemia, and signs of hyperestrogenism, such as anovulatory uterine bleeding, infertility, late onset of menopause, and hyperplasia of the stroma of the ovaries with associated endometrial hyperplasia. Endometrioid endometrial carcinoma is estrogen-responsive, and the main risk factor for this disease is long-term exposure to excess endogenous or exogenous estrogen without adequate opposition by a progestin [4]. These patients mainly have well or moderately differentiated tumors, superficial invasion of the myometrium, high sensitivity to progestins, and a favorable prognosis (85% 5-year survival rate) [5].

Type II endometrial carcinomas tend to present at an advanced stage and develop without previous hyperplasia. These non-estrogen-related carcinomas including serous adenocarcinoma, tend to be poorly differentiated and clinically more aggressive. Approximately 70% of patients with uterine serous carcinoma, some of them serous papillary (UPSC), and 50% with clear cell carcinomas present with stage III or IV disease. The patients who fall in this pathogenic group tend to have poorly differentiated tumors, deep myometrial invasion, a high frequency of metastatic disease to the lymph nodes, decreased sensitivity to progestin, and poor prognosis (58% 5-year survival rate) [6].

2 Endometrial Hyperplasia

Endometrial hyperplasia is rare in women under the age of 30 with an increasing incidence with age and an overall peak incidence of 386/100,000 women in women aged 50–54 years. The incidence then appears to decrease, with endometrial hyperplasia being found to be more common in early postmenopausal women (within 5 years of menopause) compared to late postmenopausal women (over 5 years from menopause) [7].

There are currently two systems of nomenclature for endometrial cancer precursors, the 1994 World Health Organization (WHO94) classification and the endometrial intraepithelial neoplasia (EIN) system. The International Society of Gynecological Pathologists (ISGyP) and International Federation of Gynecology and Obstetrics (FIGO) used a classification system of endometrial hyperplasia that divided it into four categories, based on architectural structure and cytologic features: simple or complex endometrial hyperplasia, with or without atypia. When the abbreviation AEH is used, it refers to atypical endometrial hyperplasia (AEH). The presence of atypia appeared to be the most important criterion for progression to adenocarcinoma or the coexistence of endometrioid adenocarcinoma. The rates of coexisting endometrioid adenocarcinoma with AEH are reported to be as low as 13% and as high as 43% [8]. More recently, four tier classification was replaced by a two tier classification. Terms "simple" and "complex" were discarded, and endometrial hyperplasia is classified into two categories, "with" or "without atypia," according to the presence or absence of atypia.

In hyperplasia without atypia, glands are crowded with very little endometrial stroma and a complex gland pattern and out-pouching formations. The incidence of simple hyperplasia is highest in women aged 50–54 years with a rate of 142/10,000 women. The natural history of hyperplasia without atypia is likely to follow a benign course. It is often seen in women near menopause when anovulatory cycles are common. The removal of the estrogenic stimulation or treatment with progestogens favorably influences the outcome. The majority of lesions will regress (60%) without treatment, and 84% will regress with progestin therapy.

Atypical hyperplasia refers to hyperplasia that contains glands with cytologic atypia and is considered premalignant. There is an increase in the nuclear/cytoplasmic ratio with irregularity in the size and shape of the nuclei. Rates of atypical hyperplasia are highest in an older population with a peak incidence of 54/100,000 women in women aged 60–64 years. This appears to correlate with a similar age of peak incidence in endometrial cancer. Atypical hyperplasia has a 36% progression rate, and even with progestins, 27% have been reported to progress to malignancy. Fifty-five percent of cases of atypical hyperplasia are expected to regress with progestin therapy. Adenocarcinomas arising or associated with atypical hyperplasia are usually of endometrioid type [9, 10].

2.1 Endometrial Intraepithelial Neoplasia Classification

The endometrial intraepithelial neoplasia (EIN) classification system was proposed by an international group of gynecologic pathologists in 2000. For a diagnosis of EIN to be made, the following criteria must be met: area of glands exceeds the stroma, cytology differs between the crowded focus and the normal background endometrium, the size of the lesion exceeds 1 mm, and benign pathology with overlapping features such as polyps or effects of exogenous estrogen can be eliminated. EIN is a precursor of type I endometrial carcinoma, which comes to clinical attention in early stages, being symptomatic. EIN must be distinguished from EIC (endometrial intraepithelial carcinoma). While EIN originates in hyperplastic endometrium, in the presence of hyperestrogenic states (endogenous or exogenous), EIC arises de novo, in atrophic endometrium (relationship with estrogen, endogenous or exogenous, still unknown), and is the precursor of type II endometrial carcinomas, with aggressive behavior.

2.2 Clinical Presentation and Diagnostic Evaluation

Endometrial hyperplasia typically presents with abnormal uterine bleeding and is most common in women who are perimenopausal or early postmenopausal. Among premenopausal women, obesity, polycystic ovarian syndrome, and chronic anovulation are common risk factors. Occasionally, in women with no abnormal uterine bleeding, endometrial hyperplasia is detected via abnormal glandular or endometrial cells on cervical cytology. Premenopausal women with irregular vaginal bleeding and postmenopausal women with any vaginal bleeding should be evaluated with an office endometrial sampling or a D&C. The gold standard for diagnosis of endometrial hyperplasia is endometrial biopsy. Most commonly this is undertaken during hysteroscopy to visualize the endometrial cavity [11].

2.3 Management

The management of endometrial hyperplasia is determined by clinical factors and by the diagnostic classification. Classification is based upon histologic features and risk of progression to endometrial carcinoma. Treatment is dependent on cause, malignant potential, fertility requirements, and medical co-morbidities as well as patient preference. Treatment options include surveillance, progestin therapy, or hysterectomy. Hormonal management of endometrial hyperplasia is recommended for those women who are not fit for surgery, for women who wish to preserve fertility, and for women with hyperplasia without atypia. All management strategies should also be accompanied by removal of the extrinsic or intrinsic source of unopposed estrogen, since excess exposure to estrogen is the main cause of endometrial neoplasia. A diagnostic D&C can also be therapeutic, and progestins or a combination of oral contraceptive agents will likely be effective. Gonadotropin-releasing hormone (GnRH) agonists, ovulation induction (e.g., with clomiphene or aromatase inhibitors), metformin, and danazol can be used as alternative to progestin treatment. The endometrium needs to be reevaluated histologically, by office biopsy or D&C, at approximately 3–6 month intervals for at least 1–2 years (see Fig. 1) [12].

Patients with endometrial hyperplasia with atypia have a high risk of progression to endometrial carcinoma and a potential for concurrent invasive disease. If atypia is present, the risk of finding an adenocarcinoma in the hysterectomy specimen ranges from 14 to 57%. The definitive treatment for complex atypical endometrial hyperplasia is hysterectomy. Surgical options include abdominal and minimally invasive procedures such as laparoscopy. ACOG does not recommend supracervical procedures as treatment because these procedures can leave behind residual disease [13].

Progestin therapy is a reasonable option for women who wish to preserve fertility or who cannot tolerate surgery [14]. Megestrol 160 mg/day, in divided doses, has been the drug of choice with acceptable results even in the face of complex endometrial hyperplasia with atypia (Fig. 2) [15].

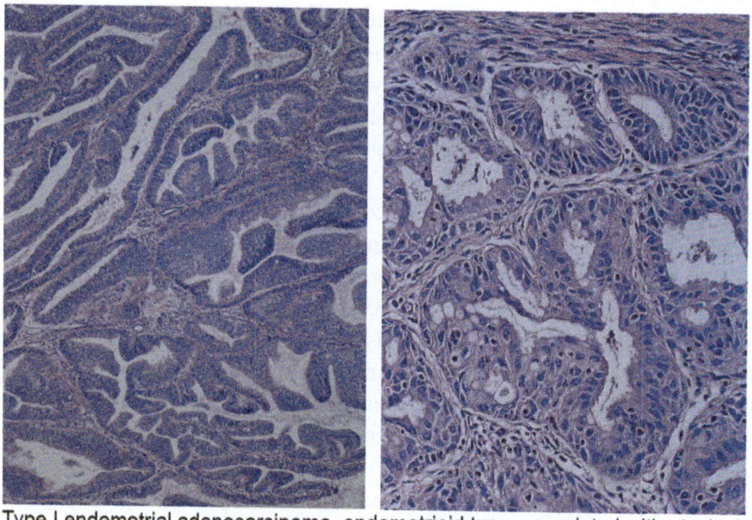

Fig. 1 Type I endometrial adenocarcinoma, endometrioid type, associated with atypical glandular (adenomatous) hyperplasia

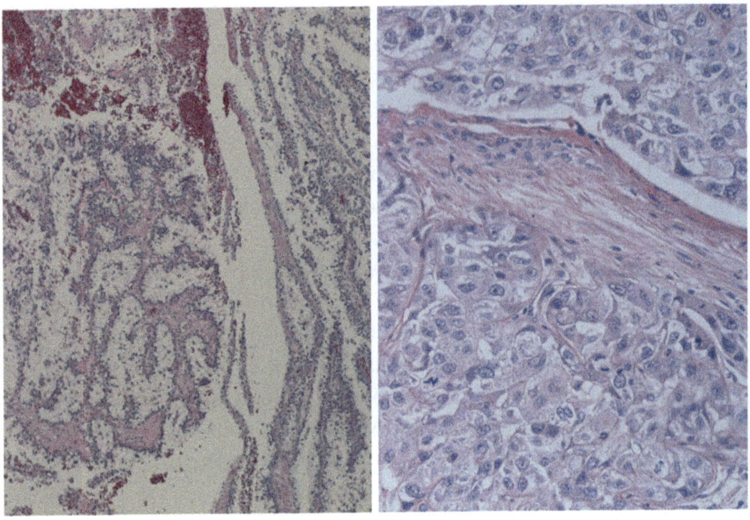

Fig. 2 Type II endometrial adenocarcinoma, clear cell (left) and serous type (right), arising in atrophic endometrium

3 Endometrial Carcinoma

Endometrial carcinomas can be classified into different histologic types (Table 1). Adenocarcinomas arising from hyperplastic endometrium or associated with atypical hyperplasia are more commonly of endometrioid type. For this histologic subtype, the median age at diagnosis is 65 years. Seventy-five percent of all uterine cancers are histologically endometrioid adenocarcinoma. For most patients with endometrioid-type tumors, particularly grade 1 or 2 lesions, and hyperplasia, hyperestrogenism is the etiologic basis [2, 9].

Adenocarcinomas are further categorized by depth of invasion and grade. The International Federation of Gynecology and Obstetrics (FIGO) uses a combination of architectural patterns and nuclear features for histologic grading [5].

The grade of an endometrial cancer endometrioid type is determined by the microscopic architectural pattern as well as the nuclear features. Architectural grade refers to the percentage of solid components found in the tumor: grade 1 (well differentiated) has less than 5% solid components, grade 2 (intermediate differentiation) has 6–50% solid components, and grade 3 (poorly differentiated) has more than 50% solid components.

Although this system relies predominantly on the glandular architecture, the most recent revision of the FIGO (International Federation of Gynecology and Obstetrics) staging system and the WHO histopathologic classification of uterine carcinoma recommend that tumors be graded using both architectural and nuclear criteria. FIGO rules for grading state that notable nuclear atypia, inappropriate for

Table 1 Classifications of endometrial carcinomas

• Endometrioid carcinoma
Squamous differentiation
Villoglandular
Secretory
• Mucinous carcinoma
• Serous endometrial intraepithelial carcinoma
• Serous carcinoma
• Clear cell carcinoma
• Neuroendocrine tumors
– Low-grade neuroendocrine tumor
Carcinoid tumor
– High-grade neuroendocrine tumor
Small cell neuroendocrine carcinoma
Large cell neuroendocrine carcinoma
• Mixed cell adenocarcinoma
• Undifferentiated carcinoma
• Dedifferentiated carcinoma

architectural grade, raises the grade of a grade 1 or grade 2 tumor by one. The grade of tumors that are architecturally grade 1 or 2 should be increased by one grade in the presence of "notable" nuclear atypia, defined as grade 3 nuclei.

By convention, serous and clear tumors are considered grade 3 or high-grade tumors.

Multiple prognostic factors have been identified for endometrial carcinoma. Histologic differentiation, stage of disease, myometrial invasion, peritoneal cytology, and lymph node metastasis are considered as important ones.

The histologic type of the endometrial carcinoma is related to prognosis, with the best prognosis associated with endometrioid adenocarcinomas, as well as better differentiated tumors with squamoid metaplasia, and secretory carcinomas. Endometrioid grade 1 and 2 tumors represent ~80% of endometrial carcinomas. These tumors usually have a favorable prognosis, are estrogen-related, and may be preceded by an intraepithelial neoplasm (atypical endometrial hyperplasia) (Fig. 1).

Poor prognostic histologic types are serous carcinomas, clear cell carcinomas, and poorly differentiated carcinomas with or without squamous elements (adenosquamous carcinoma), as previously noted. These tumors usually present as grade 3 tumors which account for 10–20% of endometrial carcinomas (Fig. 2) [16].

Higher-grade tumors are associated with increased incidence of lymph node metastasis, myometrial invasion, and a poorer overall prognosis. For staging purposes, FIGO classifies depth of invasion as less than 50% of the myometrium or greater than 50% of the myometrium. [17].

3.1 Staging, Prognosis with Risk Factors

Tumor stage is a well-recognized prognostic factor for endometrial carcinoma (Table 2). Careful evaluation of the endometrial lining by the pathologist is essential for proper diagnosis and treatment of endometrial cancer [18].

Because of the considerable discrepancy between the clinical extent of disease spread and pathologic spread noted after surgical staging, FIGO adopted a surgical-pathologic staging classification in 1988. FIGO staging classification attempts to categorize patients into prognostic groups based on extent of disease and tumor grade (Table 3) [5].

Older patients have tumors of a higher stage and grade when compared to younger patients [19]. White patients have a higher survival rate than black patients, a finding partially explained by higher-stage and higher-grade tumors among black women. In addition, black women are more likely to develop uterine serous cancers.

The clinical determinants are patient age at diagnosis, race, and clinical tumor stage. The pathologic determinants are tumor grade, histologic type, tumor size, depth of myometrial invasion, microscopic involvement of vascular spaces in the uterus by tumor, and spread of tumor outside the uterus to the retroperitoneal lymph nodes, peritoneal cavity, or uterine adnexa.

One of the most important prognostic factors for uterine cancer is the presence of extrauterine disease. The lymph node assessment in patients with early-stage disease is controversial. The rate of nodal involvement varies with stage and histology. Whereas well-differentiated tumors with superficial invasion have a 3–5% risk of nodal metastasis, deeply invasive poorly differentiated tumors have up to a 20% risk of nodal involvement. High-grade histology, such as serous or clear cell tumors, is also associated with increased risk of nodal metastasis. Myometrial invasion greater than one-half and tumors larger than 2 cm are also associated with an increased risk of nodal disease [20].

As mentioned earlier, endometrioid endometrial carcinoma is estrogen-responsive, and the main risk factor for this disease is long-term exposure to excess endogenous or exogenous estrogen without adequate opposition by a progestin.

Table 2 Five-year survival based on FIGO 2009 staging criteria; staging in these patients includes lymphadenectomy

FIGO stage	Five-year overall survival, %
IA	90.3%
IB	80.8%
II	80.5%
IIIA	68.5%
IIIB	53.1%
IIIC1	58.3%
IIIC2	51.2%
IVA	22.0%
IVB	21.1%

Table 3 International Federation of Gynecology and Obstetrics 2009 staging for endometrial carcinoma

Stage	
IA	Tumor confined to uterine corpus, <50% myometrial invasion
IB	Tumor confined to uterine corpus, ≥50% myometrial invasion
II	Tumor invades cervical stroma but confined to uterus
IIIA	Tumor invades uterine serosa or adnexa
IIIB	Involvement of vagina or parametrium
IIIC1	Metastasis to pelvic lymph nodes
IIIC2	Metastasis to para-aortic lymph nodes
IVA	Invasion of bladder or bowel mucosa
IVB	Distant metastases including intra-abdominal metastasis, inguinal lymph nodes, or both

Hormone replacement therapy (oral, patch, vaginal ring with systemic dose) with estrogen without an opposing progestin in a woman with a uterus results in a markedly increased risk of endometrial hyperplasia or carcinoma. The risk is related to both estrogen dose and duration of use. Despite the risk of unopposed estrogen, women who develop endometrial cancer appear to have favorable prognostic factors. Stage of disease and histologic grade appear to be lower in estrogen users. The poor prognostic subtypes, such as serous adenocarcinoma, clear cell carcinoma, and adenosquamous carcinoma, appear less frequently in estrogen users. As a result, survival rates with estrogen-related endometrial cancer are much better than those of non-estrogen-related cancers. The risk of endometrial hyperplasia and carcinoma with estrogen therapy can be significantly reduced by the concomitant administration of a progestin. This was first illustrated by the Women's Health Initiative randomized trial, which compared continuous estrogen-progestin therapy with placebo. Women who used oral contraceptives at some time in their life had decreased risk of developing endometrial cancer compared with women who had never used oral contraceptives. This protection occurred in women who used oral contraceptives for at least 12 months, and protection continued for at least 10 years after oral contraceptive use [21, 22].

Tamoxifen is a nonsteroidal, synthetic triethylene estrogen derivative used in the adjuvant therapy of breast cancer and also prophylactic. It induces binding to the estrogen receptors in the nuclear DNA resulting in a decrease of the unbound receptors available. It acts as an estrogen antagonist on the breast tissue, but on the uterus, tamoxifen is both agonistic and antagonistic to estrogens, especially in postmenopausal patients. During tamoxifen therapy, more so in prolonged administration of the drug, numerous patients developed endometrial polyps and myometrial leiomyomas and adenomyosis. Most endometrial polyps are benign, displaying often mucinous metaplasia and stromal fibrosis; occasional malignant changes are associated with benign cystic polyps. High-grade malignant tumors such as malignant mixed Müllerian tumors and high-grade endometrial adenocarcinomas have been reported [23–26]. In the largest published series studying endometrial tissue from

700 patients treated with tamoxifen for breast cancer, high-grade endometrial cancer was more common (2/3 vs. 1/3) than low-grade endometrioid carcinomas usually seen in hyperestrogenic patients. Most patients, however, had benign endometrial biopsies showing cyclic changes, atrophy, and benign polyps in 24%. Malignant changes were seen mostly in the polyps, more frequently in older patients, with longer duration of tamoxifen therapy [27]. Despite the undesirable effects of this therapy on the uterus, it is now considered that the benefits (prevention of contralateral breast cancer, recurrence, beneficial effects on the cardiovascular and skeletal systems) exceed the deleterious effects of tamoxifen therapy in breast cancer patients. Early diagnosis of endometrial malignancy is possible with hysteroscopy, ultrasound examination, and endometrial biopsies.

3.2 Diagnosis

Abnormal uterine bleeding is the most common clinical presentation in women diagnosed with endometrial carcinoma. Occasionally, women with no abnormal uterine bleeding present with abnormal findings on cervical cytology. Type II endometrial carcinoma not associated with endometrial hyperplasia may present with late-stage vaginal bleeding.

The risk of endometrial carcinoma and the need for endometrial evaluation depend on age, symptoms, and the presence of risk factors. The amount of bleeding does not correlate with the risk of cancer. All postmenopausal women with uterine bleeding must be evaluated for endometrial cancer, although only 20% of these patients will have a malignant genital neoplasm.

If endometrial carcinoma is found, endocervical curettage may be performed to rule out invasion of the endocervix. A routine cytologic examination (Pap smear) from the exocervix, which screens for cervical neoplasia, detects endometrial carcinoma in only approximately 50% of the cases [28–30].

3.3 Hormone Receptors

3.3.1 Estrogen

Endometrial cancer is strongly influenced by hormonal factors, with established risk factors including obesity, menstrual and reproductive changes, and exogenous hormones. Estrogens play a mitogenic role in the normal endometrium, stimulating tissue growth during the first part of the menstrual cycle. The risk of endometrial hyperplasia and cancer with unopposed estrogen therapy is both duration- and dose-dependent. Creasman and associates noted that in stage I and stage II cancers, progesterone receptor-positive status was a highly significant, independently prognostic factor in endometrial cancer. Although estrogens appeared to influence both type I and II tumors, studies showed that the association of unconjugated estradiol was stronger for the type I tumors, consistent with a central role for estrogens in influencing the progression of endometrial hyperplasias to these malignancies. The relative risk of endometrial cancer increased by estrogen therapy, and the excess risk persisted 5 or more years after cessation of therapy; however, the tumors that develop may be less aggressive as survival is better in women with cancers associated with estrogen therapy [2, 7].

Studies have shown that unconjugated estradiol is more strongly linked to low-grade than to high-grade tumors, which supports the data suggesting that the high-grade endometrioid tumors may be etiologically distinct from type I cancers and more resemble type II cancers [2].

3.3.2 Progesterone

Progesterone inhibits estrogen-induced endometrial growth during the luteal phase, while also transitioning the endometrium to a receptive state that is ready for blastocyst implantation. This balance between pro-growth estrogens and anti-growth progestogens is often dominated by estrogens during cancer development.

In the subset of patients with type I endometrial cancer who are either unable to undergo surgery or want to maintain fertility, progestins (synthetic progestogens) are given as the main course of treatment. Progestins work by binding to and activating progesterone receptor (PR). Progestins are generally well tolerated. Side effects are usually minor and include weight gain, edema, thrombophlebitis, headache, and occasional hypertension. In patients with medical comorbidities, use of hormonal agents may be preferable to cytotoxic chemotherapy. Current recommendations for progestin therapy include oral medroxyprogesterone acetate (Provera), intramuscular medroxyprogesterone acetate (Depo-Provera), and megestrol acetate (Megace) [31, 32, 38].

3.4 Management

3.4.1 Surgical Approaches

Surgery with hysterectomy and salpingo-oophorectomy is the mainstay of management of endometrial cancer. Laparoscopy has been associated with fewer postoperative complications than laparotomy. Most patients who have endometrial cancer will have stage I endometrial carcinoma. Need for further treatment is based on intraoperative and histologic findings [33].

Pelvic and para-aortic lymphadenectomy remain controversial; practice varies across different institutions or surgeons. There is yet no consensus about which patients will require lymph node staging. Sentinel lymph node evaluation following lymphatic mapping has become a standard option for the management of the retroperitoneal lymph nodes in endometrial cancer. Data supporting the use of sentinel lymph node dissection include prospective and retrospective studies showing increased detection of lymph node metastasis and a low false-negative rate compared with systematic lymph node dissection [34].

3.4.2 Chemotherapy and Hormone Therapy

Cytoreduction therapy (debulking with surgery and chemotherapy or radiation) appears to improve overall survival rates in patients with intra-abdominal disease, also decreasing recurrence rates. More favorable results using paclitaxel with and without carboplatin have been demonstrated. Evidence to support the use of adjuvant progesterone therapy to prevent endometrial cancer recurrence is lacking. Progesterone is a treatment option for patients with stage I endometrial cancer who wish to preserve fertility.

There is a 30% chance that the patient whose biopsy showed a grade 1 carcinoma may have a grade 2 or 3 carcinoma diagnosed in the hysterectomy specimen; this can be explained by the heterogeneity in tumor differentiation. Discordance between the curettage and hysterectomy specimens occurs in 15–25% of the cases [35]. Patients should be counseled on immediate hysterectomy once childbearing is completed. There are a number of tumor characteristics that increase the likelihood of response to hormone therapy. These include low-grade tumors, the presence of steroid hormone receptors, and a longer disease-free interval [36].

3.4.3 Radiotherapy

Radiation therapy is an option for patients who are medically inoperable. Postoperative brachytherapy for endometrial cancer consists of the placement of an applicator within the vaginal cavity to irradiate very focally the vaginal vault and the upper 2–3 cm of the vaginal cavity to a depth of 5 mm. The objective is to potentially sterilize residual cells in the vaginal vault and to avoid a vaginal recurrence. Because the irradiated volume is very small and the total dose is relatively low, this treatment is usually very well tolerated with only minor and transient acute side effects (proctitis, cystitis, vaginal discharge). External beam radiation therapy has decreased pelvic recurrences compared with vaginal vault brachytherapy alone but yielded no survival benefit and impaired quality of life and global health status [37].

References

1. Sponholtz T, Palmer J, Rosenberg L, Hatch E, Adams-Campbell L, Wise L. Reproductive factors and incidence of endometrial cancer in U.S. black women. Cancer Causes Control. 2017;28(6):579–88.

2. Setiawan V, Yang H, Pike M, McCann S, Yu H, Xiang Y, Wolk A. Type I and II endometrial cancers: have they different risk factors? J Clin Oncol. 2013;31(20):2607–18.
3. Deligdisch L, Marin T, Melana S, Mandel J, Holland JF, Pogo B. Human mammary tumor virus (HMTV) in endometrial carcinoma. Int J Gynecol Cancer. 2013;23:1423–8.
4. Bokhman J. Two pathogenetic types of endometrial carcinoma. Gynecol Oncol. 1983;15:10.
5. Lewin S, Herzog T, Barrena MN, Deutsch I, Burke W, Sun X, Wright J. Comparative performance of the 2009 international federation of gynecology and obstetrics' staging system for uterine corpus cancer. Obstet Gynecol. 2010;116(5):1141–9.
6. Grice J, Ek M, Greer B, Koh W, Muntz H, Cain J, Tamimi H, Stelzer K, Figge D, Goff B. Uterine papillary serous carcinoma: evaluation of long-term survival in surgically staged patients. Gynecol Oncol. 1998;69(1):69–73.
7. Damle R, Dravid N, Suryawanshi K, Gadre A, Bagale P, Ahire N. Clinicopathological Spectrum of endometrial changes in peri-menopausal and post-menopausal abnormal uterine bleeding: a 2 years study. J Clin Diagn Res. 2013;7(12):2774–6.
8. Kendall B, Ronnett B, Isacson C, Cho K, Hedrick L, Diener-West M, Kurman R. Reproducibility of the diagnosis of endometrial hyperplasia, atypical hyperplasia, and well-differentiated carcinoma. Am J Surg Pathol. 1998;22:1012.
9. Deligdisch L, Cohen CJ. Histologic correlates and virulence implication of endometrial carcinoma associated with adenomatous hyperplasia. Cancer. 1985;56:1452.
10. Fox H, Buckley C. The endometrial hyperplasias and their relationship to endometrial neoplasia. Histopathology. 1982;6:493.
11. Emons G, Beckmann M, Schmidt D, P. Mallmann and Uterus commission of the Gynecological Oncology Working Group (AGO). New WHO classification of endometrial hyperplasias. Geburtshilfe Frauenheilkd. 2015;75(2):135–6.
12. Gallos I, Ganesan R, Gupta J. Prediction of regression and relapse of endometrial hyperplasia with conservative therapy. Obstet Gynecol. 2013;121(6):1165–71.
13. ACOG Practice Bulletin. Management of endometrial cancer. Obstet Gynecol. 2005;65.
14. Gal D, Edman C, Vellios F, Forney J. Long-term effect of megestrol acetate in the treatment of endometrial hyperplasia. Am J Obstet Gynecol. 1983;143(3):316–22.
15. Cade T, Quinn M, Rome R, Neesham D. Progestogen treatment options for early endometrial cancer. BJOG. 2010;117(7):879–84.
16. Kurman R, Carcangiu M, Herrington C, R. E. Young and World Health Organization. WHO classification of tumours of the female reproductive organs. 2014. pp. 126–50.
17. Brinton L, Felix A, McMeekin D, Creasman W, Sherman M, Mutch D, Cohn D, Walker J, Moore R, Downs L, Soslow R, Zaino R. Etiologic heterogeneity in endometrial cancer: evidence from a Gynecologic Oncology Group trial. Gynecol Oncol. 2013;129(2):277–84.
18. Creasman W, DeGeest K, DiSaia P, Zaino R. Significance of true surgical pathologic staging: a Gynecologic Oncology Group study. Am J Obstet Gynecol. 1999;181:31–4.
19. Deligdisch L, Kase NG, Bleiweiss IJ. Endometrial cancer in elderly women: a histologic and steroid receptor study. Gerontology. 2000a;46:17–21.
20. Vargas R, Rauh-Hain J, Clemmer J, Clark R, Goodman A, Growdon W, Schorge J, Del Carmen M, Horowitz N, Boruta DN. Tumor size, depth of invasion, and histologic grade as prognostic factors of lymph node involvement in endometrial cancer: a SEER analysis. Gynecol Oncol. 2014;133(2):216–20.
21. Creasman W. Estrogen replacement therapy: is previously treated cancer a contraindication? Obstet Gynecol. 1991;77(2):308–12.
22. Creasman W, Henderson D, Hinshaw W, Clarke-Pearson D. Estrogen replacement therapy in the patient treated for endometrial cancer. Obstet Gynecol. 1986;67(3):326–30.
23. Dieudonne AS, Lambrechts D, Smeets D, Belmans A, Wildiers H, Paridaens R, Hyonil C, Timmerman D, Christiaens MR, Vergote I, Neven P. The rs1800716 variant in CYP2D6 is associated with an increased double endometrial thickness in post-menopausal women on tamoxifen. Ann Oncol. 2014;25:90–5.

24. Hrstka R, Podhorec J, Nenutil R, Sommerova L, Obacz J, Durech M, Faktor J, Bouchal P, Skoupilova H, Vojtesek B. Tamoxifen-dependent induction of AGR2 is associated with increased aggressiveness of endometrial Cancer cells. Cancer Investig. 2017;35:313–24.
25. Magriples U, Naftolin F, Schwartz PE, Carcangiu M. High-grade endometrial carcinoma in tamoxifen-treated breast cancer patients. J. Clin Oncol. 1993;11:485–90.
26. Robinson DC, Bloss JD, Schiano MA. A retrospective study of tamoxifen and endometrial cancer in breast cancer patients. Gynecol Oncol. 1995;59:186–90.
27. Deligdisch L, Kalir T, Cohen CJ, De Latour M, Le Bouedec G, Penault-Llorca F. Endometrial histopathology in 700 patients treated with tamoxifen for breast cancer. Gynecol Pathol. 2000b;78:181–6. Selected for Breast Diseases: A Yearbook Quarterly 2001, publ. Mosby Yearbook Inc.
28. Clark T, Barton P, Coomarasamy A, Gupta J, Khan K. Investigating postmenopausal bleeding for endometrial cancer: cost-effectiveness of initial diagnostic strategies. BJOG. 2006;113:502.
29. Dijkhuizen F, Mol B, Brölmann H, Heintz A. The accuracy of endometrial sampling in the diagnosis of patients with endometrial carcinoma and hyperplasia: a meta-analysis. Cancer. 2000;89:1765.
30. Torres M, Weaver A, Kumar S, Uccella S, Famuyide A, Cliby W, Dowdy S, Gostout B, Mariani A. Risk factors for developing endometrial cancer after benign endometrial sampling. Obstet Gynecol. 2012;120(5):998–1004.
31. Hwang J, Kim D, Bae H, Kim M, Jung Y, Yun B, Seong S, Shin E, Kim M. Combined oral medroxyprogesterone/Levonorgestrel-intrauterine system treatment for women with grade 2 stage IA endometrial Cancer. Int J Gynecol Cancer. 2017;27(4):738.
32. Park J, Kim D, Kim T, Kim J, Kim J, Kim Y, Kim Y, Bae D, Nam J. Hormonal therapy for women with stage IA endometrial cancer of all grades. Obstet Gynecol. 2013;122(1):7–14.
33. Creutzberg C, van Putten W, Koper P, Lybeert M, Jobsen J, Wárlám-Rodenhuis C, De Winter K, Lutgens L, van den Bergh A, van de Steen-Banasik E, Beerman H, van Lent M. Surgery and postoperative radiotherapy versus surgery alone for patients with stage-1 endometrial carcinoma: multicentre randomised trial. Lancet. 2000;355(9213):1404–11.
34. Khoury-Collado F, Murray M, Hensley M, Sonoda Y, Alektiar K, Levine D, Leitao M, Chi D, Barakat R, Abu-Rustum N. Sentinel lymph node mapping for endometrial cancer improves the detection of metastatic disease to the regional lymph nodes. Gynecol Oncol. 2011;122(2):251–4.
35. Obermair A, et al. Endometrial cancer: accuracy of the finding of a well differentiated tumor at dilatation and curettage compared to the findings at subsequent hysterectomy. Int J Gynecol Cancer. 1999;9:383–6.
36. Deleon M, Ammakkanavar N, Matei D. Adjuvant therapy for endometrial cancer. J Gynecol Oncol. 2014;25(2):136–47.
37. Creutzberg C, van Putten W, Koper P, Lybeert M, Jobsen J, Wárlám-Rodenhuis C, De Winter K, Lutgens L, van den Bergh A, van der Steen-Banasik E, Beerman H, van Lent M, PORTEC Study Group. Survival after relapse in patients with endometrial cancer: results from a randomized trial. Gynecol Oncol. 2003;89(2):201–9.
38. Gunderson C, Fader A, Carson K, Bristow R. Oncologic and reproductive outcomes with progestin therapy in women with endometrial hyperplasia and grade 1 adenocarcinoma: a systematic review. Gynecol Oncol. 2012;125(2):477.
39. American Cancer Society. American Cancer Society. Facts & Figures. 2019. https://www.cdc.gov/cancer/uterine/statistics/index.htm

Endometriosis and Endometriosis-Associated Ovarian Cancer (EAOC)

Tanja Pejovic, Sarah Thisted, Michael White, and Farr R. Nezhat

1 Introduction

Endometriosis is a gynecologic disease that affects over 10% of women of reproductive age causing pelvic pain, dysmenorrhea, and infertility, resulting in significant disability and reduced quality of life [1, 2].

In endometriosis the endometrial glands, stroma, and blood vessels develop outside the uterus, most commonly in the ovary, often creating cystic cavities lined by endometrial tissue (ovarian endometriotic cysts). Hormonal-related cyclic changes may involve the ectopic endometrial tissue the shedding of which may fill the closed cavity of the cyst with blood irritating the epithelial lining and producing an inflammatory reaction. The endometrioid tissue lining may also react by epithelial atypical hyperplasia and even neoplasia, in a manner somehow similar to that in the uterine cavity and under the same hormonal influences. It should be mentioned that

T. Pejovic
Department of ObGyn, Oregon Health and Science University, Portland, OR, USA

S. Thisted
University of British Columbia, Vancouver, BC, Canada

M. White
Department of Minimally Invasive Gynecologic Surgery, NYU-Winthrop University Hospital, Mineola, NY, USA

F. R. Nezhat (✉)
Department of Minimally Invasive Gynecologic Surgery, NYU-Winthrop University Hospital, Mineola, NY, USA

Nezhat Surgery for Gynecology/Oncology, New York, NY, USA

Weill Cornell Medical College of Cornell University, New York, NY, USA

Stony Brook University School of Medicine, Stony Brook, NY, USA
e-mail: farr@farrnezhatmd.com

L. Deligdisch-Schor, A. Mareş Miceli (eds.), *Hormonal Pathology of the Uterus*, Advances in Experimental Medicine and Biology 1242,
https://doi.org/10.1007/978-3-030-38474-6_5

endometriosis develops during the reproductive period of a woman's life being absent before puberty and in late menopause, except for the iatrogenic effect of hormone therapy.

The diagnosis of endometriosis requires histologic evidence of the presence of endometrial glandular and stromal tissue outside of the uterus. Microscopically, the tissue may exhibit estrogen-related changes (cell proliferation) and, during pregnancy or with progestin therapy, secretory changes and even stromal decidualization. The vicinity of steroid hormone-secreting Graafian follicles may enhance their effect on the ovarian endometriotic foci.

The most frequent sites affected by the endometriosis are the ovaries, posterior cul-de-sac, fallopian tubes, bladder, and large and small bowel, but endometriosis may affect almost any organ in the body such as the lung and even the brain.

2 Pathogenesis

Several hypotheses have been suggested as the etiology of the endometriosis. The most accepted is the theory of retrograde menstruation whereby the retrograde menstrual flow through the fallopian tubes into the peritoneal surface seeds these surfaces and organs leading to attachment of endometrial cells and their proliferation at distant pelvic and abdominal sites and peritoneal cavity. Second hypothesis, coelomic metaplasia, assumes that metaplastic changes in the peritoneum, under stimuli from the estrogen stimulation, environment, infections, or other agents, transform the mesothelium into endometrial cells to develop endometriosis. Very recent genetic studies have suggested that endometriosis is a clonal disease in the epithelium and its development is independent of stroma, providing new insight into the genesis of endometriosis.

3 The Relationship of Endometriosis and Ovarian Cancer

The association between endometriosis and ovarian cancer has perplexed clinicians and scientists for many years since it was first reported by Sampson in 1925 [3]. Today endometriosis is classified in typical and atypical, based on the degree of histological atypia. At the present time, it is, however, unclear if atypical endometriosis is a true precursor of endometriosis-associated ovarian cancer (EAOC) or whether it represents an inflammatory and reactive histologic background [4]. The clear cell carcinoma and endometrioid carcinoma are the most frequent histologic types associated with endometriosis; however, even serous and mucinous subtypes have been found in association with endometriosis occasionally.

Several excellent reviews have summarized the current evidence on endometriosis and EAOC including theories on possible pathogenesis of ovarian cancer arising from endometriosis, yet to date there is no clear mechanism and uniform hypothesis that would explain the risk of ovarian cancer in women with endometriosis and the etiology of EAOC.

The significance of this relationship was reported by Britton in a large Swedish study of 20,686 women hospitalized because of endometriosis and followed for 11.4 years and is further confirmed by Brinton et al. in 2004 with a retrospective cohort study conducted in the United States [5], analyzing the correlation of endometriosis causing primary infertility and ovarian cancer, resulting in an SIR of 4.19 (95% CI 2.0–7.7) and a risk ratio of 2.72 (95% CI 1.1–6.7) compared with patients with secondary infertility and no endometriosis. Further analysis within the cohort of primary infertility patients with endometriosis in 2005 by Brinton et al. again revealed elevated relative risks (95% CI) of 2.9 (1.2–7.1) for ovarian cancer, 2.4 (0.7–8.4) for colon cancer, 4.65 (0.8–25.6) for thyroid cancer, and 2.3 (0.8–6.7) for melanomas [6]. These Swedish cohort studies were expanded by Melin et al. in 2006 to evaluate whether risk ratios were consistent with longer follow-up [7]. The cohort was 64,492 endometriosis patients discharged from hospitalization identified through the Swedish Inpatient Registry from 1969 to 2000. When cross-referenced with the national Swedish Cancer Registry, 3349 patients were identified to have developed ovarian cancer. With extended follow-up and calculation of updated standardized incidence ratios, there was no risk for overall cancer (1.04), but an increase was noted in ovarian cancer (1.43 [95% CI 1.2–1.7]), endocrine tumors (1.36 [95% CI 1.2–1.6]), non-Hodgkin lymphoma (1.24 [95% CI 1.0–1.50]), and brain tumors (1.22 [95% CI 1.0–1.4]). Importantly, the risk for women with early diagnosis and long-standing endometriosis was most pronounced, with standardized incidence ratios (SIRs) of 2.01 and 2.23, respectively [8]. Of note, women with a history of hysterectomy at or before time of endometriosis diagnosis did not show an elevated risk [9]. Again, both studies of the Swedish cohorts may be skewed to reflect malignant incidence ratios for cases of more severe endometriosis, because the cohorts were hospitalized patients with more advanced stages of endometriosis. Also, because records of hospitalized patients were retrospectively cross-referenced with a separate cancer patient registry, there is the possibility of negating or including cases erroneously.

Olsen et al. completed the largest study that did not support the increased ovarian cancer risk in endometriosis patients [9]. Analyzing a group of 37,434 postmenopausal women, a cohort of 1392 postmenopausal patients who self-reported the diagnosis of endometriosis was isolated. After an average 13-year follow-up, no significant increased risk was found for all cancers, breast cancer, or ovarian cancer, but there was a significant association with increased risk of non-Hodgkin lymphoma, with an age-adjusted risk ratio of 1.8 (95% CI 1.0–3.0). This study involved acceptable long-term follow-up; however, several factors must be taken into account. The study was underpowered, as the cohort was smaller and included only three ovarian cancer cases. Furthermore, the endometriosis was not histologically confirmed, and, because all of the patients were postmenopausal, it is possible that younger patients may have already developed ovarian cancer and died. Table 1 summarizes the epidemiologic studies of ovarian cancer risk in endometriosis patients.

Table 1 Epidemiologic studies assessing ovarian cancer risk in endometriosis patients

Author	Study type	Cohort size	Mean follow-up (years)	Ovarian malignancies identified	Ovarian cancer in endometriosis patients (SIR/OR)	
Brinton et al., 1997 [19]	Cohort	20,686 endometriosis patients	11.4	29	Overall cancer risk	
					Ovarian cancer	1.2
					Ovarian cancer with ≥10 years	1.9
					Follow-up	2.5
					Ovarian cancer with long-standing endometriosis	4.2
Brinton et al., 2004 [20]	Cohort	12,193 infertility patients		45	Ovarian cancer	2.5
Brinton et al., 2005 [5]	Cohort			2491	2.53 (1.19–5.38)	
Ness et al., 2000 [17]	Case control			66	Ovarian cancer	1.7
Borgfeldt and Andolt 2004 [19]	Nested case control	28,163		81	Ovarian cancer	1.3
Modugano et al., 2006 [21]	Case control			177	1.3 (1.1–1.6)	
Melin et al., 2006 [7]	Cohort	64,492	12.7	122	Overall cancer risk	1.04
					Ovarian cancer	1.43
					Ovarian cancer early	2.0
					Diagnosed endometriosis	2.2
					Ovarian cancer with long-standing endometriosis	
Olson et al., 2002 [8]	Cohort	1392	13	3	No increased risk for overall or ovarian cancer	
Kobayashi et al., 2007 [22]	Cohort	6398	12.8	46	Ovarian cancer	8.95
					Ovarian cancer >50 years old	13.2

Reciprocal analysis of the prevalence of endometriosis found in ovarian cancer patients also supports the clinical correlation. In a review of 29 studies from 1973 to 2002 on the prevalence of endometriosis in epithelial ovarian cancers organized by location of disease, the following three groups were compiled: (1) histologic proof of transition from ovarian endometriosis to cancer as defined by Sampson [10], (2) ovarian cancers with endometriosis in the same ovary, and (3) ovarian cancers with concomitant pelvic endometriosis. The second category was considered to be the best estimation of endometriosis in the different histologic subtypes, yielding a prevalence of 4.5% in serous, 1.4% in mucinous, 35.9% in clear cell, and 19% in endometrioid carcinomas [11, 12].

These data were further corroborated by Valenzuela et al. in 2007 [13]; among 22 cases of ovarian endometrioid adenocarcinomas of the ovary, three patients were found to have concomitant endometriosis as defined by the Sampson criteria. The review by Van Gorp et al. calculated an ovarian cancer prevalence of 0.9% in all cases of endometriosis, 2.5% when present in the same ovary, and 4.5% when coexistent with any pelvic endometriosis [11]. Malignant extraovarian endometriosis is estimated to account for 25% of all malignant transformations of endometriosis and 80% of the endometrioid subtype [14–16].

Looking at the trend of ovarian cancer in endometriosis is more difficult because endometriosis is not always aggressively resected and confirmed by histopathologic studies. Only a limited number of the studies controlled for confounding factors for both diseases, such as parity, infertility, tubal ligation, ovarian hyperstimulation, and duration of endometriosis; Ness et al. completed two case–control studies confirming the association between endometriosis and ovarian cancer [17, 18]. In a group of 767 women with ovarian cancer and 1367 control subjects, with adjustments made for age, parity, family history of ovarian cancer, race, oral contraceptive use, tubal ligation, hysterectomy, and breast-feeding, overall women with breast cancer were 1.7-fold more likely to report an endometriosis history [17]. Furthermore, in a pooled study of 13,000 women, ovarian cancer was more likely among subfertile women, especially with infertility resulting from endometriosis, showing an odds ratio of 1.9 (95% CI 1.2–2.9) [18].

In 2012, Pearce et al. suggested that ovarian cancer risk associated with endometriosis varies according to histologic subtype of ovarian cancer [23]. In a pooled analysis of 13 case–control studies from the Ovarian Cancer Association Consortium database, the investigators assessed self-reported endometriosis data from a total of 23,144 women—13,326 controls, 7911 with invasive ovarian cancer, and 1907 with borderline ovarian cancer. When stratified by age (5-year categories) and ethnic origin (non-Hispanic white, Hispanic white, black, Asian, and other) and adjusted for duration of oral contraceptive use (ranging from 0 to ≥10 years), self-reported history of endometriosis was associated with a significantly increased risk of invasive clear cell, invasive low-grade serous, and invasive endometrioid ovarian cancer subtypes. No association was found between a history of endometriosis and invasive mucinous, invasive high-grade serous, or borderline (both serous and mucinous) ovarian cancer [23, 24].

Over the last few years, a new paradigm for ovarian cancer pathogenesis has emerged that presupposes two distinct types of ovarian epithelial carcinoma with distinct molecular profiles: type I and type II carcinomas. Type I tumors include endometrioid, clear cell carcinoma, and low-grade serous carcinoma and mostly arise via defined sequence either from endometriosis or from borderline serous tumors, mostly presenting in an early stage. Histologic evidence of endometriosis is found in 23–36% of type I endometrioid and clear cell ovarian cancers [25]. Together these cancers are known as endometriosis-associated ovarian cancer (EAOC). In a clinical and histological correlation study of endometriosis and ovarian cancer [26], out of 76 with stage 1 invasive ovarian cancer, ovarian endometrioma was present in 40 cases. Fifty-four patients had non-serous carcinomas (40 endometrioid, 10 clear, and 4 mixed endometrioid and clear cell carcinoma), and all had ovarian endometriomas, peritoneal endometriosis, or both. Interestingly, one third had abnormal endometrial pathology such as endometrioid adenocarcinoma, hyperplasia, or polyp. No serous carcinoma patient presented with pelvic pain and abnormal vaginal bleeding with or without pelvic pain [26].

The type II serous carcinomas, which overall represents the bulk of ovarian malignancies, were not associated with pelvic endometriosis.

Recent molecular studies in type I ovarian carcinomas identified the presence of somatic mutations in *ARID1A*, *KRAS*, *PTEN*, *PIK3CA*, *MLH1*, and B catenin [27, 28]. In addition, *TP53*, *BCL2*, and *POLE* mutations have also been described [29, 30].

Similar gene mutations have been found both in EAOC and adjacent benign endometriosis suggesting that they share the common clonal origin [31]. PTEN mutation were found in benign endometriotic cysts as well as in endometrioid and clear cell ovarian carcinoma suggesting that PTEN may be involved early in malignant transformation of endometriosis. On the other hand, in EAOC, KRAS mutation is frequently seen in endometrioid and mucinous carcinomas, but it is not present in adjoining endometriosis or atypical endometriosis.

ARID1A is a tumor suppressor gene that encodes BAF250a protein, a member of SWI/SNF chromatin remodeling complex [32]. Mutations in *ARID1A* have been found in clear cell carcinoma (46–95%) and in endometrioid carcinoma of the ovary (30%) [33]. The high frequency of *ARID1A* mutation, leading to a functional loss of the protein, strongly suggests its role in EAOC.

TP53 mutation which is otherwise pathognomonic for high-grade serous ovarian carcinoma is found in 30% of endometriosis when it is associated with clear cell carcinoma. Benign endometriosis has not been associated with *TP53* mutation, and it has not been found in endometriosis coexisting with endometrioid carcinoma (reviewed in [4]).

4 Epigenetics

The role of epigenetic gene regulation in endometriosis and EAOC is currently under investigation. The exact mechanism and the interrelation of multiple epigenetic changes are not fully understood, yet it is known that EAOC despite sharing in general common genetic aberration does behave different biologically; this may be a consequence of epigenetic gene silencing or activation. The two main types of EAOC, clear cell carcinoma (CCC) and endometrioid cancer (EC), have different biomarkers. Transcription factor HNF1β (hepatocyte nuclear factor-1β) *is* a biomarker of ovarian CCC histology, but not of EC. HNF1β-positive cells have been found both in clear cell carcinoma and adjacent endometriosis. The main role of HNF1β is in glycogen synthesis, antioxidative defense, anti-apoptosis, and resistance to chemotherapy. HNF1β is overexpressed in clear cell carcinoma whereby it upregulated glycolysis and yielded increased amount of lactate. This allows cancer cells to avoid excess reactive oxygen species (ROS) production, thereby allowing survival advantage in endometrioma. On the other hand, HNF1β upregulates the synthesis of glutathione and antioxidant, and that gain also gives advantage to clear cell carcinoma survival.

EC has a high expression of estrogen receptors ERα and ERβ. This expression is significantly higher than in clear cell carcinoma (reviewed in [34]). Estrogen receptor expression may be modifiable by a number of facts such as epigenetic (methylation, acetylation) or heme binding. In endometriosis ERβ is hypomethylated, and therefore the protein is overexpressed, while ERα is lower in endometriosis [35]. Upregulation of ER and hyperestrogenic state may lead to malignant transformation into EC in endometriosis, not associated with clear cell carcinoma. Overexpression of ER is actually associated with better outcome of both EC and CCC, not having a role in cancer progression [36]. Further, hypomethylation of ER gene promoter is correlated with *HNF1β* gene promoter hypermethylation in EC [37]. The combination of low ER and high HNF1β is a potential marker of EC.

5 The Role of Microenvironment and Immune System

Endometriosis is a chronic inflammatory condition, and endometriotic cells are adaptable to microenvironment with high levels of cytokines and heme, initially. However, the interplay between these factors and endometriotic cells may start the cascade of cellular events eventually leading to remodeling of extracellular matrix and malignant transformation [38]. Several molecules have been reported as crucial in this process such as MMP-2 as well as CXCR4 which increases VEGF and stimulates the process of angiogenesis in endometriotic foci [39, 40].

The theory of the so-called redox imbalance has been out forward recently to unify different factors involved in the pathogenesis of endometriosis and associated cancers. In this hypothesis, repeated episodes of retrograde menstruation lead to bleeding into endometriotic cysts and pelvic cavity and release of hemoglobin (Hob), free iron, and heme. Persistent exposure to high heme concentrations exposes tissues to high oxidative stress and formations of reactive oxidative species (ROS). ROS promote DNA damage and early carcinogenesis. It is important to know that most of the iron in endometriotic cyst is heme iron, and not free iron. Heme iron is oxidized to metHb with generation of superoxide anion 02—via antioxidation. The levels of nitric oxide which catabolizes the reaction from oxyHb to metHb is elevated in serum and peritoneal fluid of the patients with endometriosis. It is metHb that induces the production of free radicals, which damage DNA. However, seemingly paradoxically, metHb is downregulated in EAOC, which shows that disturbed balance between oxidative stress and antioxidants is in favor of antioxidants in EAOC (reviewed in [34]). Therefore, this concept of malignant transformation of endometriosis proposes that iron metabolism involvement in malignant transformation of endometriosis is a two-step process: first the by-products of heme metabolism induce ROS and oxidative stress, and then synthesis of antioxidants occurs with consequent resistance to apoptosis and tumor initiation (reviewed in [34]).

While scientists are on the tract to identify the molecular pathways involved in endometriosis and EAOC, the very critical clinical question remains as on how to identify women with endometriosis who are at risk of developing EAOC based on the current knowledge.

Although ovarian cancer will develop in only 0.3–1.6% of women with endometriosis, it is important to assess, document, and systematically follow up the risk factors that may predispose patients to developing ovarian cancer. These include the following: (1) long-standing endometriosis, (2) endometriosis diagnosed at an early age, (3) endometriosis associated with infertility, and (4) the presence of enlarging ovarian endometrioma or changing characteristics and mural nodule formation.

Women found to be at an increased risk of ovarian endometrioma have options of medical (hormonal) or surgical treatment. The treatment should be personalized based on patient's age, desire for childbearing, family history, and type and characteristics of endometriomas. Nezhat et al. have described two types of endometriomas: type I and type II [41].

Type I endometriomas are characterized by small lesions that spread across peritoneal and ovarian surfaces, whereas type II endometriomas originally start as functional hormone-secreting ovarian cysts that are invaded by cortical endometriosis and gradually develop into endometriomas. Hormonal treatment often results in incomplete regression of endometriotic lesions and recurrence of endometriomas. Additionally, in type II endometriomas, adjuvant hormonal suppressive therapy that prevents ovulation can decrease the risk of recurrent ovarian endometrioma formation [41]. Melin et al. showed that women who underwent unilateral oophorectomy for endometriosis had a significantly reduced risk of later development of ovarian cancer, with an OR of 0.19 (95% CI, 0.08–0.46) compared with controls. In addition, ovarian cancer was significantly less likely to develop in women who underwent radical surgical excision of all visible endometriosis, with an OR of 0.30 (95% CI, 0.12–0.74) [42].

In light of the accumulated data and observations regarding endometriosis and ovarian cancer, criteria may be established to stratify the risk of cancer by identifying and monitoring women with endometriosis for risk factors and pursuing risk-reducing medical and surgical treatment options in these women. At the time of surgical diagnosis and treatment, consideration for complete resection of pelvic endometriosis, salpingectomy, oophorectomy, or hysterectomy should be individualized based on a patient's age, desire for future fertility, and preoperative consultation with the patient [43]. These initiatives, if validated, should substantially reduce the risk of ovarian cancer as well as the total mortality risk. As new research becomes available, the recommendations may be refined in terms of both screening and prevention.

In addition to ovarian endometriosis, extraovarian endometriosis may also be associated with malignant transformation (i.e., bowel, bladder, cesarean section scars) [44, 45]. The review by Van Gorp et al. [10] shows ovarian cancer to be prevalent in 0.9% of all endometriosis cases. Furthermore, it shows 2.5% prevalence when present in the same ovary and 4.5% when coexistent with pelvic endometriosis. It is estimated that malignant extraovarian endometriosis accounts for 25% of all malignant endometriosis transformations, 80% of which are of the endometrioid cancer subtype [45]. This rate of incidence of non-ovarian endometriosis transformation suggests that a more in-depth focus on this issue is necessary. There are also reported cases of synchronous endometriosis-associated ovarian and endometrial cancers in certain patient populations.

6 Synchronous Endometrial Carcinoma with Endometrioid Ovarian Carcinoma

Although the association between endometriosis and some subtypes of ovarian cancer has been well established, there is less known about the association between endometriosis and endometrial cancer. More evidence is showing patients with a history of endometriosis that are presenting with synchronous endometrioid endometrial carcinomas (EEC) and endometrioid ovarian carcinomas (EOC). The rate of endometrial cancer diagnosis was significantly higher in women with endometriosis and EOC (33%) than in other ovarian malignancies (11%) (p = 0.04) [46, 47]. Deligdisch et al. (2007) retrospectively reviewed 76 patients with stage 1 ovarian carcinoma and histologic characteristics. Forty patients had a diagnosis of EOC with endometriosis, and 17/40 (22%) of patients had coinciding endometrial cancer or 11/40 (14%) with endometrial hyperplasia or polyps [48]. In an earlier study of endometrial cancer, Walsh et al. discovered that at time of surgery, 25% of patients with known endometrial carcinoma were found to have also ovarian carcinoma, >90% EOC [49]. Evidence from molecular studies by Schultheis et al. (2016) demonstrated that 17 patients who underwent genome sequencing had similarities in genetic mutations in EECs and EOCs. Interestingly, four patients had bilateral

EOCs and EEC which were found to be all clonally related [47]. Anglesio et al. showed that there is a clear genetic relationship between EOC and endometriosis [50]. There is no clear evidence of the pathogenesis for these findings; however there are several theories. It can be hypothesized that endometrial cells, migrating into the pelvis with the retrograde menstruation, can give rise to atypical endometriosis and to EAOC [51]. Another hypothesis is that synchronous endometrial and ovarian (SEO) carcinomas result from the dissemination of cells from one organ site to another. However, whether this can be considered a metastasis, dissemination, or the same mutation that occurs in both tissues remains unclear [51]. Most patients with simultaneous EOC and endometrial neoplasia display an analogous hyperestrogenic hormonal profile [26].

7 Treatment for EAOC

After primary staging and debulking surgery, there are no established guidelines for the management of a patient with endometriosis-associated ovarian carcinoma (EAOC). Depending on histologic type and disease stage, treatments are varied from expectant management, adjuvant chemotherapy, radiation therapy, or a combination approach due to the rarity of disease [52–57]. EAOC have mostly two main histologic subtypes: clear cell carcinoma (CCC) and endometrioid carcinoma (EC) [58]. Several population-based studies compared outcomes of patients with prior endometriosis with diagnosed CCC and EC versus patients without endometriosis. EAOC patients were diagnosed at a younger age, had earlier stage of disease, had decreased recurrence rates (26.9% vs. 41%), and had an improved overall 5-year survival (75% vs. 55%) [56, 58–60].

Early-stage disease CCC and EC treated with adjuvant chemotherapy was shown to decrease disease recurrence. Regimens mainly consisted of carboplatin/paciltaxel or irinotecan/cisplatin for 6 cycles in retrospective cohort studies [61–63]. This was beneficial for stage 1C yet controversial for stages 1A and 1B with lower recurrence rates and no significant difference in overall survival [64–66]. Later stages of CCC have shown resistance to chemotherapy, whereas chemotherapy for EC should remain with standard regimens [61, 62].

Later-stage CCC treated with radiotherapy has shown improved survival and decreased mortality in several studies likely due to its resistance to standard chemotherapy regimens. Nagai et al. (2007) treated patients with external beam radiotherapy versus platinum chemotherapy for stages 1–3. Results showed an increase in disease-free survival and overall survival (81.2% and 81.8%, respectively) in the radiation group versus 25.0% and 33.3% in the platinum group [67]. Swenerton et al. (2010) treated patients with adjuvant radiotherapy having a 40% reduction in disease-specific mortality [68]. Hoskins et al. (2012) treated patients with combination carboplatin/paclitaxel and radiation with an improved disease-free survival of 20% at 5 years [69].

Endocrine therapy for treatment of endometriosis has been previously studied to decrease symptoms and potential progression of disease after surgical treatment [70–73]. These hormonal treatments are also well documented in the treatment of endometrial carcinoma especially for premenopausal patients seeking future fertility [74, 75]. For both CCC and EC, there is evidence for the use of adjuvant treatment with aromatase inhibitors or progesterone [76, 77]. Several studies and phase II trials utilized aromatase inhibitors specifically with recurrent EC or chemotherapy-resistant EC with decreased rates of recurrence and increased survival [78–80]. Initial data for adjuvant aromatase inhibitors and progesterone treatments used as a long-term maintenance therapy have also been promising [43, 81, 82].

8 Conclusion

Although not yet fully delineated, there is a strong relationship between endometriosis, ovarian cancer, and some endometrial cancers. Gynecologists as well as general practitioners must be mindful of the apparently increased risk of ovarian cancer among endometriosis patients. Special attention should be paid to patients with early endometriosis diagnosis, a long-standing history of disease, associated infertility, and/or infertility treatment, as these patients seem to be at the highest risk. Advancements in more precise diagnostic analysis into the pathogenesis of endometriosis and the possibility of malignant transformation may help to provide new insights into diagnostic and treatment modalities. Specifically, further elucidation of the involved genetic and immune mechanisms of endometriosis is necessary. Overall, once the transition from benign endometriosis to atypical and malignant tissue is clearly elucidated, marker expression can be analyzed to guide clinical management and outcome. Genomics and proteomics may facilitate the development of these diagnostic and therapeutic tools. At this time, however, surgical resection followed by medical treatment remains the primary method of treatment of endometriosis. With the correlation of endometriosis and ovarian cancer continuing to strengthen over time, appropriate and timely resection and elimination of disease should be practiced.

References

1. Eskenazi B, Warner ML. Epidemiology of endometriosis. Obstet Gynecol Clin N Am. 1997;24(2):235–58.
2. Lim MC, et al. Clinical presentation of endometrioid epithelial ovarian cancer with concurrent endometriosis: a multicenter retrospective study. Cancer Epidemiol Biomark Prev. 2010;19(2):398–404.
3. JA S. Endometrial carcinoma of ovary arising in endometrial tissue in that organ. Arch Surg. 1925;10:1–72.
4. Kajiyama H, et al. Endometriosis and cancer. Free Radic Biol Med. 2019;133:186–92.

5. Brinton LA, et al. Causes of infertility as predictors of subsequent cancer risk. Epidemiology. 2005;16(4):500–7.
6. Melin A, et al. Endometriosis and the risk of cancer with special emphasis on ovarian cancer. Hum Reprod. 2006;21(5):1237–42.
7. Melin A, Sparen P, Bergqvist A. The risk of cancer and the role of parity among women with endometriosis. Hum Reprod. 2007;22(11):3021–6.
8. Olson JE, et al. Postmenopausal cancer risk after self-reported endometriosis diagnosis in the Iowa Women's Health study. Cancer. 2002;94(5):1612–8.
9. Kondi-Pafiti A, et al. Clinicopathological characteristics of ovarian carcinomas associated with endometriosis. Arch Gynecol Obstet. 2012;285(2):479–83.
10. Van Gorp T, et al. Endometriosis and the development of malignant tumours of the pelvis. A review of literature. Best Pract Res Clin Obstet Gynaecol. 2004;18(2):349–71.
11. Brinton LA, et al. Cancer risk after a hospital discharge diagnosis of endometriosis. Am J Obstet Gynecol. 1997;176(3):572–9.
12. Valenzuela P, et al. Endometrioid adenocarcinoma of the ovary and endometriosis. Eur J Obstet Gynecol Reprod Biol. 2007;134(1):83–6.
13. Heaps JM, Nieberg RK, Berek JS. Malignant neoplasms arising in endometriosis. Obstet Gynecol. 1990;75(6):1023–8.
14. Benoit L, et al. Malignant extraovarian endometriosis: a review. Eur J Surg Oncol. 2006;32(1):6–11.
15. Modesitt SC, et al. Ovarian and extraovarian endometriosis-associated cancer. Obstet Gynecol. 2002;100(4):788–95.
16. Ness RB, et al. Factors related to inflammation of the ovarian epithelium and risk of ovarian cancer. Epidemiology. 2000;11(2):111–7.
17. Ness RB, et al. Infertility, fertility drugs, and ovarian cancer: a pooled analysis of case-control studies. Am J Epidemiol. 2002;155(3):217–24.
18. Vigano P, et al. Bias versus causality: interpreting recent evidence of association between endometriosis and ovarian cancer. Fertil Steril. 2007;88(3):588–93.
19. Borgfeldt C, Andolf E. Cancer risk after hospital discharge diagnosis of benign ovarian cysts and endometriosis. Acta Obstet Gynecol Scand. 2004;83(4):395–400.
20. Brinton LA, et al. Ovarian cancer risk associated with varying causes of infertility. Fertil Steril. 2004;82(2):405–14.
21. Modugno F, et al. Oral contraceptive use, reproductive history, and risk of epithelial ovarian cancer in women with and without endometriosis. Am J Obstet Gynecol. 2004;191(3):733–40.
22. Kobayashi H, et al. Risk of developing ovarian cancer among women with ovarian endometrioma: a cohort study in Shizuoka, Japan. Int J Gynecol Cancer. 2007;17(1):37–43.
23. Pearce CL, et al. Association between endometriosis and risk of histological subtypes of ovarian cancer: a pooled analysis of case-control studies. Lancet Oncol. 2012;13(4):385–94.
24. Ozerlat I. Gynecological cancer: Endometriosis link to invasive subtypes. Nat Rev Clin Oncol. 2012;9(4):189.
25. Wei JJ, William J, Bulun S. Endometriosis and ovarian cancer: a review of clinical, pathologic, and molecular aspects. Int J Gynecol Pathol. 2011;30(6):553–68.
26. Deligdisch L, et al. Stage I ovarian carcinoma: different clinical pathologic patterns. Fertil Steril. 2007;88(4):906–10.
27. Zou Y, et al. The presence of KRAS, PPP2R1A and ARID1A mutations in 101 Chinese samples with ovarian endometriosis. Mutat Res. 2018;809:1–5.
28. Takeda T, et al. ARID1A gene mutation in ovarian and endometrial cancers (review). Oncol Rep. 2016;35(2):607–13.
29. Ishikawa M, et al. Affinity-purified DNA-based mutation profiles of endometriosis-related ovarian neoplasms in Japanese patients. Oncotarget. 2018;9(19):14754–63.
30. Nezhat F, et al. Comparative immunohistochemical studies of bcl-2 and p53 proteins in benign and malignant ovarian endometriotic cysts. Cancer. 2002;94(11):2935–40.

31. Anglesio MS, et al. Cancer-associated mutations in endometriosis without cancer. N Engl J Med. 2017;376(19):1835–48.
32. Munksgaard PS, Blaakaer J. The association between endometriosis and ovarian cancer: a review of histological, genetic and molecular alterations. Gynecol Oncol. 2012;124(1):164–9.
33. Wiegand KC, et al. ARID1A mutations in endometriosis-associated ovarian carcinomas. N Engl J Med. 2010;363(16):1532–43.
34. Kobayashi H, et al. Integrating modern approaches to pathogenetic concepts of malignant transformation of endometriosis. Oncol Rep. 2019;41(3):1729–38.
35. Bukulmez O, et al. Inflammatory status influences aromatase and steroid receptor expression in endometriosis. Endocrinology. 2008;149(3):1190–204.
36. Rambau P, et al. Association of hormone receptor expression with survival in ovarian endometrioid carcinoma: biological validation and clinical implications. Int J Mol Sci. 2017;18(3):515.
37. Yamaguchi K, et al. Epigenetic determinants of ovarian clear cell carcinoma biology. Int J Cancer. 2014;135(3):585–97.
38. Kobayashi H, et al. Novel biomarker candidates for the diagnosis of ovarian clear cell carcinoma. Oncol Lett. 2015;10(2):612–8.
39. Jana S, et al. Regulation of matrix metalloproteinase-2 activity by COX-2-PGE2-pAKT axis promotes angiogenesis in endometriosis. PLoS One. 2016;11(10):e0163540.
40. Del Carmen MG, et al. Endometriosis-associated ovarian carcinoma: differential expression of vascular endothelial growth factor and estrogen/progesterone receptors. Cancer. 2003;98(8):1658–63.
41. Nezhat F, et al. Clinical and histologic classification of endometriomas. Implications for a mechanism of pathogenesis. J Reprod Med. 1992;37(9):771–6.
42. Melin AS, et al. Hormonal and surgical treatments for endometriosis and risk of epithelial ovarian cancer. Acta Obstet Gynecol Scand. 2013;92(5):546–54.
43. Nezhat FR, et al. New insights in the pathophysiology of ovarian cancer and implications for screening and prevention. Am J Obstet Gynecol. 2015;213(3):262–7.
44. Nezhat F, et al. The relationship of endometriosis and ovarian malignancy: a review. Fertil Steril. 2008;90(5):1559–70.
45. Nezhat CH, et al. Laparoscopic management of 15 patients with infiltrating endometriosis of the bladder and a case of primary intravesical endometrioid adenosarcoma. Fertil Steril. 2002;78(4):872–5.
46. Mangili G, Bergamini A, Taccagni G, Gentile C, Panina P, Viganò P, et al. Unraveling the two entities of endometrioid ovarian cancer: a single center clinical experience. Gynecol Oncol. 2012 Sep;126(3):403–7.
47. Schultheis AM, et al. Massively parallel sequencing-based Clonality analysis of synchronous endometrioid endometrial and ovarian carcinomas. J Natl Cancer Inst. 2016;108(6):djv427.
48. Deligdisch L, et al. Stage I ovarian carcinoma: different clinical pathologic patterns. Fert Stert. 2006;88(4):906–10.
49. Walsh, et al. Coexisting ovarian malignancy in young women with endometrial cancer. Obstet Gynecol. 2005 Oct;106(4):693–9.
50. Anglesio MS, et al. Multifocal endometriotic lesions associated with cancer are clonal and carry a high mutation burden. J Pathol. 2015;236:201–9.
51. Garavaglia, et al. The origin of endometriosis-associated ovarian cancer from uterine neoplastic lesions. Med Hypoth. 2018;110:80–2.
52. Matias-Guiu X, Stewart CJ. Endometriosis-associated ovarian neoplasia. Pathology. 2018;50(2):190–204.
53. Yu HC, et al. Increased association between endometriosis and endometrial cancer. A nationwide population based retrospective cohort study. Int J Gynecol Cancer. 2015;25(3):447–52.
54. Poole EM, et al. Endometriosis and risk of ovarian and endometrial cancers in a large prospective cohort of U.S. nurses. Cancer Causes Control. 2017;28(5):437–45.
55. Worley MJ, et al. Endometriosis associated ovarian cancer: a review of pathogenesis. Int J Mol Sci. 2013;14:5367–79.

56. Barreta A, et al. Endometriosis associated ovarian cancer: population characteristics and prognosis. Int J Gynecol Cancer. 2018;28(7):1251–7.
57. Noli S, et al. Long term survival of ovarian endometriosis associated clear cell and endometrioid ovarian cancers. Int J Gynecol Cancer. 2013;23(2):244–8.
58. Nagar H, et al. Adjuvant pelvic radiation therapy +/− vaginal brachytherapy in patients with high risk stage I or stage II uterine papillary serous, clear cell, and high-grade endometrioid carcinoma. Am J Clin Oncol. 2016;39(4):335–9.
59. Davis M, et al. Comparison of clinical outcomes of patients with clear cell and endometrioid ovarian cancer associated with endometriosis to papillary serous carcinoma of the ovary. Gynecol Oncol. 2014;132(2):760–6.
60. Paik ES, et al. Clinical outcomes of patients with clear cell and endometrioid ovarian cancer arising from endometriosis. J Gynecol Oncol. 2018;29(2):e18.
61. Sahin H, et al. Is the presence of endometriosis associated with a survival benefit in pure ovarian clear cell carcinoma? Arch Gynecol Obstet. 2018;297(4):1005–13.
62. Bell J, et al. Randomized phase III trial of three versus six cycles of adjuvant carboplatin and paciltaxel in early stage epithelial ovarian carcinoma: a gynecologic oncology group study. Gynecol Oncol. 2006;102(3):432–9.
63. Chan JK, et al. The potential benefit of 6 vs 3 cycles of chemotherapy in subsets of women with early stage high risk epithelial ovarian cancer: an exploratory analysis of a gynecologic oncology group study. Gynecol Oncol. 2010;116(3):301–6.
64. Takano M, et al. Clear cell carcinoma of the ovary: a retrospective multicentre experience of 254 patients with complete surgical staging. Brit J Cancer. 2006;94(10):1369–74.
65. Shu CA, et al. Ovarian clear cell carcinoma, outcomes by stage: the MSK experience. Gynecol Oncol. 2015;139(2):236–41.
66. Sugiyama T, et al. Randomized phase III trial of irinotecan plus cisplatin compared with paclitaxel plus carboplatin as first line chemotherapy for ovarian clear cell carcinoma: JGOG3017/GCIG trial. J Clin Oncol. 2016;34(24):2881–7.
67. Nagai Y, et al. Postoperative whole abdominal radiotherapy in clear cell adenocarcinoma of the ovary. Gynecol Oncol. 2007;107:469–73.
68. Swenerton KD, et al. Histotype predicts the curative potential of radiotherapy: the example of ovarian cancers. Ann Onc. 2010;22(2):341–7.
69. Hoskins PJ, et al. Low stage ovarian clear cell carcinoma: population based outcomes in British Columbia Canada, with evidence for a survival benefit as a result of irradiation. J Clin Oncol. 2012;30(14):1656–62.
70. Winkler UH, Ferguson H, Mulders JA. Cycle control, quality of life and acne with two low-dose oral contraceptives containing 20 microg ethinylestradiol. Contraception. 2004;69(6):469–76.
71. Witjes H, Creinin MD, Sundström-Poromaa I, Martin Nguyen A, Korver T. Comparative analysis of the effects of nomegestrol acetate/17 β-estradiol and drospirenone/ethinylestradiol on premenstrual and menstrual symptoms and dysmenorrhea. Eur J Contracept Reprod Health Care. 2015;20(4):296–307.
72. Muzii L, Di Tucci C, Achilli C, et al. Continuous versus cyclic oral contraceptives after laparoscopic excision of ovarian endometriomas: a systematic review and metaanalysis. Am J Obstet Gynecol. 2016;214(2):203–11.
73. Casper RF. Progestin-only pills may be a better first-line treatment for endometriosis than combined estrogen-progestin contraceptive pills. Fertil Steril. 2017;107(3):533–6.
74. Staubhar A, et al. Successful treatment of low-grade endometrial cancer in premenopausal women with an aromatase inhibitor after failure with oral or intrauterine progesterone. Gynecol Oncol Rep. 2017;10(21):10–2.
75. Jerzak K, et al. Endocrine therapy in endometrial cancer: an old dog with new tricks. Gynecol Oncol. 2019;153(1):175–83.
76. Pedernea E, Gomora M, Morales-Vasquez F, Perez-Montiel D, Mendez C. Progesterone reduces cell survival in primary culture of endometrioid ovarian carcinoma. J Ovarian Res. 2019;12(1):15–22.

77. Bowman A, et al. CA125 response is associated with estrogen receptor expression in a phase II trial of letrozole in ovarian cancer: identification of an endocrine sensitive subgroup. Clin Cancer Res. 2002;8:2233–9.
78. Papadimitriou CA, et al. Hormonal therapy with letrozole for relapsed epithelial ovarian cancer. Long term results of a phase II study. Oncology. 2004;66:112–7.
79. Smyth JF, et al. Antiestrogen therapy is active in selected ovarian cancer cases: the use of letrozole in estrogen receptor positive patients. Clin Cancer Res. 2007;13:3617–22.
80. Ramirez PT, et al. Efficacy of letrozole in the treatment of recurrent platinum and taxane resistant high grade cancer of the ovary or peritoneum. Gynecol Oncol. 2008;110:56–9.
81. Zhao D, et al. Prognostic role of hormone receptors in ovarian cancer: a systematic review and meta-analysis. In J Gynecol Cancer. 2013;23(1):25–33.
82. Modungo F, et al. Contraceptive use, reproductive history, and risk of epithelial ovarian cancer in women with and without endometriosis. Am J Obstet Gynecol. 2004;191(3):733–44.

Hormone Therapy in Menopause

John Paciuc

1 Introduction

Menopause is by definition the final menstrual period (FMP) resulting from marked decrease in ovarian estrogen production confirmed by 12 months of amenorrhea [1]. In natural menopause, the mean age is 52, with a wide range of 40–58. As women frequently live past 80, a third of their lives will be spent in menopause and beyond [1, 2]. The low estrogen levels of the menopause transition often trigger bothersome systemic vasomotor symptoms (VMS) and night sweats and, over time, equally bothersome local symptoms of vulvovaginal atrophy (VVA) and dyspareunia and other urogenital symptoms, now termed genitourinary syndrome of menopause (GSM).

Menopausal hormone therapy (MHT), previously referred to as hormone replacement therapy (HRT), is FDA approved and endorsed by North American Menopause Society (NAMS), the International Menopause Society (IMS), and the Endocrine Society for use, where there are no contraindications, for four indications:

1. Vasomotor symptoms (VMS) that are bothersome
2. Osteoporosis prevention and fracture reduction (in postmenopausal women)
3. Genitourinary syndrome of menopause (GSM)
4. Premature ovarian insufficiency (POI) and Early natural menopause

MHT is either in the form of estrogen (ET) alone for women without a uterus or as a combination of estrogen–progestogen (EPT) for women with a uterus. The indication for progestogen use is to prevent endometrial hyperplasia or endometrial cancer from unopposed estrogen. Progestogens are a large extremely heterogeneous family of steroid molecules that fall into two categories: (1) Progestins—all by definition *synthetic* such as medroxyprogesterone acetate (MPA), norethindrone acetate, and many others and (2) Progesterone —all native and *natural*.

J. Paciuc (✉)
Lenox Hill Hospital, Mount Sinai Hospital, New York, NY, USA

L. Deligdisch-Schor, A. Mareş Miceli (eds.), *Hormonal Pathology of the Uterus*, Advances in Experimental Medicine and Biology 1242,
https://doi.org/10.1007/978-3-030-38474-6_6

2 Contraindications for MHT

In general, MHT should not be used in women with undiagnosed abnormal vaginal bleeding, known liver impairment or disease, prior estrogen-sensitive breast or endometrial cancer, personal history of thromboembolic disease such as DVT or pulmonary thromboembolism, or inherited high risk of thromboembolic disease such as known protein C, protein S, or antithrombin deficiency, active or history of thromboembolic disease such as stroke or MI or coronary heart disease, dementia/Alzheimer's disease, porphyria cutanea tarda, and hypertriglyceridemia (>400 mg/dL oral ET) [3, 4].

Caution should be exercised in women with gallbladder disease (oral route), diabetes, hypoparathyroidism (hypocalcemia risk), benign meningioma, intermediate or high risk of breast cancer, high risk of heart disease, and migraine with aura [4]. There are lesser concerns that endometriosis may reactivate and that leiomyomas may grow [3].

More common adverse effects (AEs) include nausea, bloating, weight gain, fluid retention, mood swings, and breast tenderness; these are more commonly progestogen-related and more with synthetic progestins such as MPA (commonly used in the past including the WHI but far less now) and less with micronized progesterone (more commonly used in current clinical practice).

3 Historical Overview

Over the past half century, the persona of estrogen has swung on a pendulum from hero to post-WHI villain and again now as the putative health champion.

4 Before the WHI

4.1 Observational Data

Conjugated equine estrogen (CEE), isolated from pregnant mare urine, was approved by the FDA for the relief of menopausal symptoms in 1942. The *New York Times* bestseller *Feminine Forever*, released in 1966, catalyzed the enthusiasm for estrogen as reliever of menopausal symptoms as well as harbinger of youth. Around that time, during the 1970s and early 1980s, small observational studies recorded 30–50% reductions in cardiovascular disease and all-cause mortality among postmenopausal users of estrogen versus nonusers [5–9]. In the late 1980s and early 1990s, observational studies, meta-analyses, and epidemiological studies continued to suggest that MHT reduced the risk of osteoporosis, coronary heart disease (CHD), dementia, and all-cause mortality [10–18].

MHT was actually endorsed by the American College of Physicians and recommended as a prevention strategy in 1992 [19]. Yet many critics felt these data may represent "healthy user" bias. Namely, women who choose to take MHT are healthier and have healthier lifestyles than women who do not. Only large randomized controlled trials could validate the observational suggestion that MHT prevents CHD and lowers mortality.

4.2 *The Postmenopausal Estrogen/Progestin Intervention (PEPI) Trial*

Prior to the WHI, the PEPI trial in 1991 enrolled women aged 45–64 all less than 10 years postmenopausal to participate in a 3-year RCT. They were randomized to five groups: (1) placebo (2) Conjugated equine estrogen (CEE)∗ (the most commonly used estrogen at the time) 0.625 mg/day alone (women without a uterus) (3) CEE 0.625 mg/day with medroxyprogesterone acetate (MPA)∗—most commonly used progestin at the time 10 mg/day for 12 days per 30-day cycle (4) CEE daily with MPA 2.5 mg continuously (both each day) and (5) CEE with micronized progesterone 200 mg/day for 12 days per 30-day cycle.

The study was very limited by the fact that blinding was suboptimal; symptomatic women who felt better knew they were on estrogen and those not better dropped out of the study knowing they were on placebo. Despite flaws, the study proved efficacy of estrogen for menopausal symptom relief, endometrial protection (from either progestogen), maintenance of bone density, and prevention of osteoporosis [5, 20, 21]. In fact, in 1995, the continuous combined estrogen and progestin regimen was approved by the FDA for the treatment of menopausal symptoms as well as for the prevention of osteoporosis.

4.3 *The Heart and Estrogen Replacement Study (HERS)*

In 1998, the HERS was a large randomized placebo-controlled clinical trial designed to test the next level of conventional thinking, namely, as studies (observational) suggest estrogen users have a lower incidence of coronary heart disease (CHD) than nonusers, can an RCT prove that estrogen can treat cardiovascular disease not just prevent it? The trial would be secondary prevention study of estrogen's efficacy in slowing the progression or even more ambitiously reversing disease in women with established coronary heart disease. 2763 women with coronary heart disease with a mean age of 67 were randomized to either oral CEE 0.625 mg plus MPA 2.5 mg daily or a placebo and followed for an average of 4 years. Although there were no statistically significant differences between groups with 172 women in the hormone group versus 176 in the placebo group with MI or CHD deaths, there were more CHD events in the hormone group especially during the first year of treatment than in the placebo group as well as more cases of thromboembolic events and gallbladder disease. The trial results were used as evidence against the recommendation of starting MHT for women with existing CHD as secondary prevention [22, 23]. Yet, unresolved was whether a large RCT could answer the question of the use of estrogen for primary prevention.

5 The Women's Health Initiative (WHI) Study

5.1 Intention and Design

The intent of the WHI study was, on a grand scale, to boldly ask whether estrogen can provide primary prevention of CHD not only in younger women 1–10 years postmenopausal as previously seen in observational studies and in the PEPI trials but also in women well beyond menopause. 27,000 women were enrolled. The average age was 63 and 12 years since menopause. The goal was to create three groups of women aged 50–54, 55–59, and 60–79, the first two groups were restricted to 10 and 20% of the total number of enrollees, respectively; consequently, the *older women* aged 60–79 years *dominated* as 70% of the study.

Women were randomized to either oral CEE (0.625 mg; Premarin) with oral MPA (2.5 mg) (EPT arm) versus placebo if they had a uterus or CEE alone (0.625 mg; Premarin) (ET arm) versus placebo if they had a hysterectomy. This leviathan $625 million NIH-funded study, planned to run for 8.5 years, had primary endpoints of CHD and breast cancer and secondary endpoints of stroke, pulmonary embolus, endometrial cancer, colon cancer, hip fracture, and all-cause mortality.

The combined estrogen plus progestin (EPT) arm of the trial was suddenly and prematurely halted in 2002 after an average of 5.2 years due to increased risks of coronary events, invasive breast cancer, stroke, and venous thrombo-embolism (VTE) which were felt to outweigh notable benefits of reduced hip fractures, colorectal cancer, and diabetes compared to placebo. The absolute risks of adverse events per 10,000 person years were actually 7 more cardiac events, 8 more strokes, 9 more pulmonary embolisms, 8 more breast cancers, 6 fewer colorectal cancers, 5 fewer hip fractures compared with placebo group, and *no difference in deaths compared to placebo*. This language of Absolute Risk is both user-friendly and noninflammatory, yet buried deep inside a paper which only went to press long after the media and public already got the news. Unfortunately, the news delivered to the media and public in an entirely different language; the bewildering and terrifying language of Hazard Ratios of 1.26 for breast cancer and 1.29 for coronary heart disease was not only was statistically significant but the news was grossly misinterpreted by the media, namely that women taking MHT had a 26% chance of developing breast cancer and a 29% chance of having a coronary event! [24].

The estrogen-only arm of the trial was then halted by the NIH 2 years later in 2004 and so the WHI ended due to an increased risk of stroke (HR 1.39 yet in absolute risk 12 additional cases per 10,000 woman-years compared to placebo) and a null effect on CHD. There were also fewer cases of breast cancer in the estrogen-only arm compared with the placebo arm.

5.2 *Aftermath and Clinical Consequences of the WHI "Early News"*

The fear and confusion generated by the initial reporting of the WHI data through the media sent shock waves through the medical and lay community. Women were fearful primarily of breast cancer as well as cardiac risks, and physicians were fearful of litigation. Over half of all women who had heard these early WHI findings reported that it adversely affected their use of HRT as well as their overall level of trust toward their physician's counseling regarding HRT.

As such, prescriptions for HRT plummeted by more than 70% over the subsequent 7 years after the WHI study; by 2010, HRT use fell below 5% to the U.S. population of women over 40 [25, 26]. Adverse clinical events followed in tandem with the drop in HRT use.

One large study that retrospectively reviewed medical records of a large HMO found that the post-WHI discontinuation of MHT was associated with a step-wise rate of increase of hip fractures; they paralleled declines in bone-mineral density (BMD) and progressed rapidly from a HR of 1.16 in the first year off MHT to a HR of 1.77 the fifth year off [27]. Another large study that retrospectively reviewed a large claims database from multiple healthcare plans demonstrated a significant increase in fractures among postmenopausal women in the 3 years after the WHI publication which followed a decline in use of MHT despite a concurrent increase in the use of other bone-modifying agents [28] Recall that prevention of osteoporosis and fractures was and remains one the four FDA approved indications of MHT in the United States as well as most other countries in the world.

The major harms of discontinuing the use of MHT is not limited to increased fractures. A study using collective data of 332,000 women with two million woman follow-up years from national registries of Finland highlighted significant cardiovascular risk directly related to discontinuing MHT. In the first year of discontinuing MHT, women who were under 60 had a two- to threefold increased risk of mortality from both myocardial infarction as well as from stroke compared with expected number of deaths in the age-matched general population in Finland [29].

An engaging mathematical study was performed using the post-hoc WHI 10-year follow-up data showing a 13 per 10,000 per year higher rate of mortality among hysterectomized women randomized to placebo compared with women aged 50–59 randomized to estrogen over a 10-year follow-up [30, 31]. The goal of the study was to calculate the mortality toll of estrogen avoidance in women who had hysterectomies in the United States between 2002 and 2011 as a direct result of the fear generated by the WHI initial results. When the excess mortality of 13/10,000 per year was applied to the calculated number of women who would have had a hysterectomy and the known percent decline in estrogen use for 10 years post-WHI, the avoidance of estrogen would have resulted in excess deaths anywhere between 19,000 and 92,000 [25, 30].

Another adverse post-WHI event was the proliferation of the "bioidentical hormone" market. "Bioidentical hormone" is a marketing rather than a medical term. Its marketing and sales flourished in a seller's market created by the post-WHI media scare of standard formulations. Often sold on the internet by nonphysicians, these are actually compounded products which may contain any variable combination of estrogens, progesterone, DHEA, testosterone, thyroxine, melatonin, and growth hormone. There is limited quality control regarding purity, dosing, batch-to-batch consistency, and lack of any clinical efficacy and safety data. The estrogens added may cause endometrial hyperplasia and the progesterone, if even added, may not be potent enough to inhibit proliferation of endometrium to hyperplasia or even cancer. Cases of endometrial cancer following the use of compounded HRT have been reported [32]. The most common estrogen used in the past and in the WHI was conjugated equine estrogen—derived from the urine of pregnant mares and the most common progestogen used was medroxyprogesterone acetate (MPA)—a synthetic progestin and neither remotely bioidentical. Currently, the most commonly prescribed estrogen is 17-B-estradiol and the most commonly prescribed progestogen is micronized progesterone—both although not compounded and instead FDA-approved as a result of passing safety and efficacy trials—are in fact by definition "bioidentical" and even more accurately "body-identical." This needs to be highlighted when discussing MHT with women.

5.3 WHI Late News but Good News

Several years after the sudden halt of the WHI in 2002 and its initial "bad news" particularly regarding CVD risk, a number of age-stratified post hoc studies were performed. Unlike the older women aged 60–79 which comprised 70% of the enrollees, the women aged 50–59 had actual beneficial and protective effects for CVD.

In 2007, it was reported that in the 50–59 year subgroup there was a 25% reduction in risk of CHD with EPT with a HR of 0.76 (95% CI 0.5–1.16) and that an adverse risk was null until 20 years from menopause [33, 34]. Moreover, both the WHI E/PR (HR 0.67; 95% CI, 0.43–1.04) and the WHI E trial (HR 0.70; 95% CI, 0.46–1.09) showed a 30% reduction in all-cause mortality in women aged younger than 60 years and/or less than 10 years since menopause when randomized to MHT compared with placebo [25, 34].

In 2006, Salpeter et al. [35] performed a meta-analysis on 23 RCTs with 39,049 women to look at MHT effect on CHD events (MI or cardiac death) in younger and older postmenopausal women. MHT significantly reduced events in younger women (OR 0.68 95% CI 0.48–0.96) but not in older women (OR 1.03 95% CI 0.91–1.16).

6 The Timing Hypothesis

The timing hypothesis (or early window or critical window hypothesis) quite simply states that the benefits of menopausal hormone therapy (MHT)—specifically estrogen—in preventing atherosclerosis occurs only when the therapy is initiated before advanced atherosclerosis develops. More specifically, it posits that giving exogenous estrogen to a woman soon after endogenous estrogen deficiency of menopause will have beneficial cardiovascular effects before atherosclerosis has had time to progress significantly. Conversely, if exogenous administration is significantly delayed with time allowed for the development of complicated atheromatous plaque, the effect will either be null or harmful [36].

The late Professor Thomas Clarkson DVM (1931–2015) was the first to propose the timing hypothesis with his seminal work on atherosclerosis in menopausal cynomolgus monkeys. He elegantly demonstrated that the time when hormone therapy is initiated with reference to when menopause started will determine its effect on coronary artery atherosclerosis. When estrogen was given immediately after surgical menopause (oophorectomy), coronary artery atherosclerosis was robustly reduced by 70%. In contrast, when the administration of estrogen was delayed by 2 years after oophorectomy (equivalent to 6 human postmenopausal years), there was no reduction of coronary artery atherosclerosis. Such a delay in the initiation of MHT in postmenopausal monkeys would allow the progression of atherosclerosis with plaque instability approximating the same phenomenon in humans aged 60–65 [37], the dominant group in the WHI study.

A concise summary of atherosclerosis progression as well as the effects of early versus late estrogen effects on the endothelium would help clarify the mechanics behind the timing hypothesis.

Atherosclerosis progresses from fatty streaks (plaque precursors) initially covering only 15% of the luminal surface in 70% of women by median age 35. Plaques increase in size and fibrous caps start developing through the menopause transition and early menopause. By median 55, plaques and their fibrous caps continue to grow with possible necrosis and calcifications. By median 65, plaques become increasingly complex with inflammation (within the plaques as well as the fibrous cap shoulders), worsening calcification, necrosis, and activation of metaloproteinases leading to overall plaque instability [37].

On healthy endothelium (i.e., with either no or only early-stage atherosclerosis) estrogens cause (1) vasodilatation through nongenomic rapid release of nitrous oxide (NO) as well as genomic expression of NOS genes, increased cox-2, and decreased endothelin; (2) decreased inflammation with reduced tumor necrosis factor-alpha a, decreased cell adhesion molecules, and decreased monocyte chemoattractant protein-1; and (3) overall decreased lesion progression rate via increased nitric oxide, decreased inflammatory cell adhesion, decreased platelet aggregation, decreased vascular smooth muscle cell proliferation, and decreased low-density lipoprotein (LDL) oxidation/binding [38]. By contrast, once the healthy endothelium is transformed by advanced atherosclerosis, estrogen's effects, rather than being protective and beneficial, become deleterious. The estrogen receptors have decreased expression/function and consequently there is decreased vasodilatation, increased inflammation and, via increases in matrix metalloproteinases (MMP) and increased neovascularization, there is overall increased plaque instability (Fig. 1) [38].

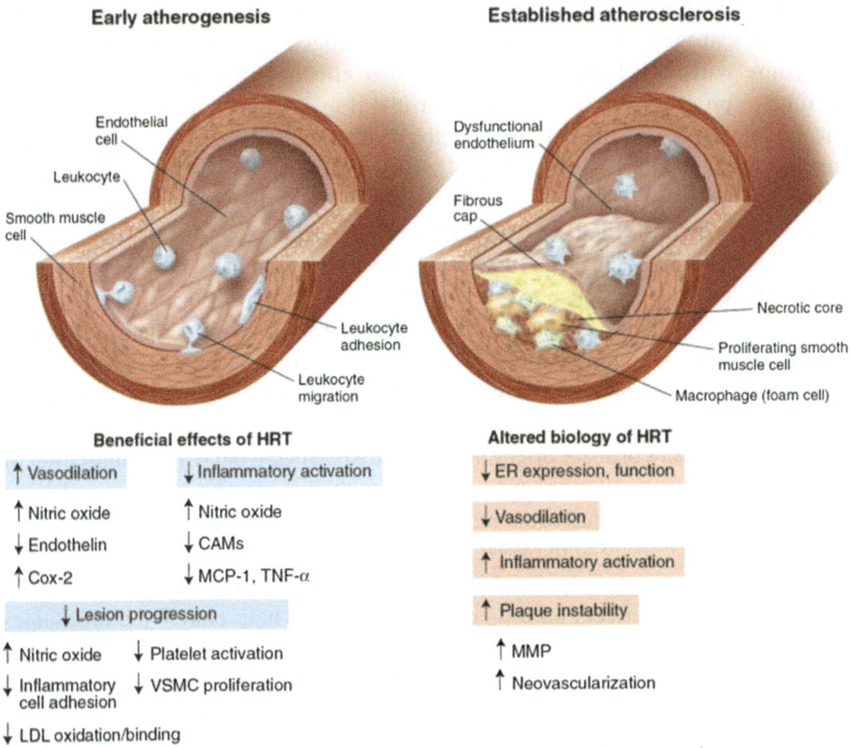

Fig. 1 The timing hypothesis: differential effects of HRT on early and later stages of atherosclerotic disease. Atherosclerosis is characterized by the gradual loss of vascular protective mechanisms and the emergence of advanced, unstable lesions [44]. SSH effects on the endothelium and its protective functions, vascular smooth muscle cells, and inflammatory cells differ, depending on the stage of atherosclerosis in the underlying blood vessel [3, 8, 23, 29, 47, 108]. *LDL* low density lipoprotein, *CAMs* cell adhesion molecules, *MCP-1* monocyte chemoattractant protein 1, *TNF-α* tumor necrosis factor–α, *VSMC* vascular smooth muscle cell, *MMP* matrix metalloproteinase, *COX-2* cyclooxygenase 2

Two clinical trials were designed specifically to test and validate the timing hypothesis: the KEEPS trial and the ELITE trial. As a moratorium was placed on government-funded HT trials after the WHI, the Kronos foundation sponsored the KEEPS (Kronos Early Estrogen Prevention Study). The KEEPS was a randomized, double-blinded placebo-controlled trial to test the hypothesis that the initiation of HT (oral conjugated equine estrogens or transdermal 17-B-estradiol) in healthy recently postmenopausal women would slow the progression of atherosclerosis by measuring changes in carotid artery intimal media thickness (CIMT). 727 women in essentially good health averaging 1.5 years postmenopause were randomized to three groups—(1) oral CEE 0.45 mg (lower than 0.625 mg dose most frequently used in clinical practice at the time of the study and also the dose used in the WHI), (2) transdermal estradiol 50 μg patches, or (3) placebo. Due to concerns over the slightly increased risk of breast cancer seen in the EP group in the WHI compared with decreased breast cancer in the E alone group, medroxyprogesterone acetate

(MPA) used in the WHI continuously in women with a uterus was replaced with micronized progesterone 200 μg 12 days each month in the KEEPS. Despite improved lipids, neither hormone formulation delayed the progression of atherosclerosis over placebo group over 4 years; specifically, the annual increases in CIMT of 0.007 mm per year was similar across all three treatment groups [39]. Although the results were surprising and could not support the timing hypothesis with its null effect, some felt this was from too low a dose of estrogen, acting on too healthy a population for too short a time. Despite this, the study confirmed in both oral and transdermal estrogen treatment arms, reductions in hot flashes, improved sleep and maintenance of bone density, and no adverse events (including venous thrombosis) [40]. An ancillary sexual function study of KEEPS [41] reported improvements in both physical and emotional domains of sexual function with both oral estrogen and transdermal estrogen arms compared with placebo. Based on completion of the well-validated Female Sexual Function Inventory (FSFI), a 19-item questionnaire covering six domains of sexual function: both physical (lubrication, pain) and emotional/libidinal (desire, arousal, orgasm, satisfaction)—the results showed similar improvement of physical symptoms of pain and lubrication with either oral or transdermal estrogen. However, with improving the libidinal domains (desire, arousal, orgasm, satisfaction), transdermal estradiol was found to be superior over oral estrogen. The explanation lies behind sex-hormone-binding globulin (SHBG) whose levels are raised by oral estrogen's hepatic first pass effect on the liver and subsequently binds up free testosterone. Less free testosterone would adversely affect libido [41]. As such, women with menopausal symptoms who also experience hypoactive sexual desire disorder (HSDD) would have another reason to benefit from transdermal over oral estrogen.

The Early Versus Late Intervention Trial (ELITE) was proposed to the NIH in 2002 to more definitively and rigorously test the timing hypothesis [42]. Six hundred and forty-three healthy postmenopausal women were stratified into two study cells according to time since menopause (1) less than 6 years (early postmenopause group) or (2) 10 or more years (late postmenopause group) and were randomized to either oral estradiol 1 mg daily plus (if with uterus) sequential 10 days of progesterone vaginal gel or oral placebo plus (if with uterus) placebo vaginal gel. The primary outcome was the rate of change of coronary artery intimal-media thickness (CIMT) which was measured every 6 months. After being followed for a median of 5 years, there was a notable difference in the effect of estradiol on CIMT progression between the early and late groups ($P = 0.007$ for the interaction). In the early group, CIMT increased by 0.0078 mm per year in the placebo group versus a slower increase by 0.0044 mm per year in the estradiol group ($P = 0.0008$).

In the late group, the rates of progression of CIMT in placebo and estradiol groups were similar (0.0088 vs. 0.0100, respectively) [42]. This study demonstrates estrogens beneficial effect on atherosclerosis progression when given early postmenopause versus a null or deleterious effect when given late and elegantly supports the timing hypothesis.

A post-trial analysis of the same ELITE trial examined the association between plasma estradiol levels and atherosclerosis progression to see if the associations were similar in both early versus late postmenopause groups. Higher serum estradiol levels were inversely associated with CIMT progression in the early group and positively associated with CIMT progression in the late group. In short, this post-trial analysis shows that the serum estradiol levels achieved with oral estradiol was associated with CIMT progression in both early and late groups but in 180° opposite directions!! To quote the investigators, "these results not only support the HT timing hypothesis tested by the main (ELITE) trial but also add an explanatory mechanism consistent with the timing hypothesis" [43].

The timing hypothesis is the final arbiter in the historical dispute over estrogen as hero versus villain and the bedrock principle supporting the main tenet of menopausal hormone therapy; namely, that when there is an indication for E or E/P, without contraindications, it should only be *initiated* in women who are younger than 60 or within the first 10 years since the onset of menopause.

6.1 Vasomotor Symptoms

Vasomotor symptoms (VMS), commonly referred to as hot flushes (or hot flashes, inferior term incorrectly implying brevity of event) and night sweats, are the hallmark symptom of menopause with an 80% prevalence. They are the most common reason for seeking medical care during the menopause transition. VMS are subjectively described as a sudden sensation of heat and warmth in the face, neck, and chest often with sweating, reddening of the skin, anxiety, palpitations, and sleep disruption. The mean duration is 3–4 min with a wide range of a few seconds to 60 min [44].

VMS can have an enormous impact on quality of life and psychosocial impairment on many levels. Their effects can run the gamut from disturbed sleep with insomnia and sleep apnea to mood swings (irritability, sadness, tension) to cognitive deficits (impaired concentration and verbal memory) to social and work impairment (disruption of family relationships, social isolation, embarrassment, anxiety, fatigue, and reduced work productivity) [44].

Long thought to be of relatively short duration, recent studies show that VMS can last over 10 years. Data from the Study of Women's Health Across the Nation (SWAN) report a median duration of 7.4 years. Four patterns or trajectories were observed:

1. The early-onset group started even before their menses stopped and waned with their final menstrual period (FMP).
2. The later-onset group started after their menses stopped and continued well into their postmenopausal years.
3. The mild vasomotor group had few or no vasomotor symptoms over the menopause transition.
4. The "Super Flasher" group—a term coined by Dr. Rebecca Thurston's lab—started their VMS before their FMP and continued well into the postmenopause for a median duration of 11.8 years (and median post FMP persistence of 9.4 years [45].

VMS are more prevalent in African-American women, those with a high BMI, less education, lower income, smoking and alcohol consumption, depression and other mood disorders, and any type of increased perceived stress and anxiety.

In a Bayesian network analysis [46] attempting to causally organize the myriad factors underlying hot flashes (HF), hormone levels of estradiol and progesterone were not surprisingly most consistently associated with HFs. Apart from hormone levels, smoking and alcohol consumption were the only other primary factors directly related with VMS. The authors further commented that the role of education as a factor might in fact be mediated by smoking as there is a strong association between education level and smoking [46].

Recent data are also reporting various forms of physical or emotional trauma as risk factors for more frequent and intense VMS. These include a history of post-traumatic stress disorder, intimate partner violence, and child abuse or neglect. One compelling study objectively showed that among a group of women reporting vasomotor symptoms, those with a physical or sexual abuse history had 1.5–2 times the number of sleep vasomotor symptoms than women without such history [47].

Lower levels of estradiol and higher levels of follicle-stimulating hormone are de facto characteristics of all menopausal women and are also consistently and repeatedly correlated to VMS [45, 46]. Yet, as not all menopausal women experience VMS, there are other partially mapped out systems that must act as facilitators [45].

6.2 Physiology of VMS

The mammalian hypothalamus maintains core temperature within a thermoneutral zone (TNZ) by effecting heat dissipation (i.e., vasodilation, sweating, cold seeking) should the core temperature rise above the TNZ and heat conservation (shivering, warm seeking behavior) and should the core temperature fall below the TNZ. The hot flush is a pathologically exaggerated heat dissipation response with peripheral vasodilatation, increased surface heat and profuse sweating with evaporative heat loss [48]. The trigger is a small elevation in core body temperature within an abnormally narrowed thermoneutral zone [48]. What causes the narrowing of the TNZ remains a puzzle; some postulate that it is declining estrogen via its association with decreased levels of endorphins and serotonin and increased levels of norepinephrine. Any medication that increases serotonin, estrogen, and endorphins or decreases norepinephrine would widen the thermoneutral zone and prevent the generation of a HF. Hence, the efficacy of SSRIs and MHT via increases of serotonin and estrogen, respectively, and of clonidine via its effect on lowering norepinephrine for treating VMS.

Although increased LH and GNRH secretion are seen with hot flushes, neither are causative. Women who lack LH from surgical removal of their pituitary can still have hot flashes from administration and withdrawal of exogenous estrogen [49, 50]. Comparably, women with Kallman's syndrome who lack hypothalamic GNRH-producing neurons can still have hot flushes with estrogen withdrawal [49, 51].

There are many neuropeptides that are implicated in the regulation of GNRH secretion: neuropeptide Y, corticotropin-releasing hormone, leptin, ghrelin, orexin A, and beta-endorphins [52]. Recent data have shown a central and dominant role of the kisspeptin/neurokinin B/dynorphin group (KNDy) of neurons, located in the hypothalamus, as the generators of the hot flush via regulation of GNRH activity. Kisspeptin acts upstream of GNRH and following stimulatory inputs from neurokinin B and inhibitory inputs from dynorphin, kisspeptin—signals directly to GNRH neurons to control GNRH pulsatile secretion [53]. Padilla et al. [54] elegantly demonstrated in the lab that direct artificial stimulation of kisspeptin neurons induced an increase in skin temperature in the tails of both female and male mice. In addition, the kisspeptin neurons became more sensitive to stimulation (activation) after ovariectomy in the female mice, suggesting that hot flush susceptibility may be altered in estrogen withdrawal states such as menopause. Attention has been drawn more specifically to neurokinin B (NKB) and its receptor neurokinin B-3 receptor (NK3R) both expressed by kisspeptin neurons to signaling hot flushes. An experiment in which premenopausal women were given NKB peripherally developed hot flushes precisely mimicking those seen in postmenopausal women [55]. A population-based study showed that SNP gene mutations in TACR3—the gene that expresses NK3R—could be linked with the variability in hot flushes experienced by postmenopausal women [55, 56].

To prove the concept that NK3R antagonism may in fact block the generation of hot flushes, Prague et al. [57] performed a randomized, double-blinded, placebo-controlled crossover trial of an oral NK3R antagonist (MLE4901). The recruited subjects, postmenopausal women with at least 7 bothersome hot flushes/24 h, were each treated for 4 weeks with agent and then another 4 weeks with placebo with a 2-week "wash-out" period in between. Both subjective reporting as well as objective measures (skin conductance) demonstrated a 73% reduction in hot flush (HF) frequency that started as soon as day 3 and lasted the full 4 weeks on the oral NK3R antagonist. In the placebo group, by contrast there was only a 28% reduction in HF frequency, similar to the 25% average placebo effect seen in other studies. This was a phase II trial and so far no products of this class have yet come to market. Their potential for improving QOL for millions of women with VMS who cannot take estrogen is enormous.

7 Treatment of VMS

7.1 Estrogen Therapy

Estrogen therapy, with or without progesterone and compared with other pharmacologic or alternative therapies, remains the most effective therapy for treating VMS [3]. In a large meta-analysis of 21 RCTs, compared with placebo, estrogen alone or combined with a progestogen reduced symptom frequency by 77% as well as symptom severity [58]. An exhaustive database search performed by NAMS found no other pharmacological or alternative therapy capable of providing more relief [3]. When MHT is discontinued, VMS will return to approximately half of women [3, 59, 60].

7.2 Nonhormonal Pharmacologic (Prescription) Therapies

7.2.1 Paroxetine

Paroxetine (Paxil), a selective serotonin reuptake inhibitor (SSRI) is the ONLY non-hormonal pharmaceutical approved by the FDA for the treatment of moderate to severe VMS. Unlike the higher dosing range of 20–50 mg/day for its usual treatment of major depressive disorders, a low dose paroxetine salt of 7.5 mg/day or standard paroxetine 10–25 mg/day is the recommended dosing for moderate to severe vasomotor symptoms alone [61, 62].

Other SSRIs and SNRIs (Selective Norepinephrine Reuptake Inhibitors) similar to paxil have proven efficacy at reducing VMS frequency and severity by placebo-controlled RCTs include escitalopram, citalopram, venlafaxine, and desvenlafaxine [61]. Contraindications to SSRIs and SNRIs include simultaneous use of monoamine oxidase (MAO) inhibitors, history of neuroleptic syndrome from prior use of antipsychotic therapy, and prior history of serotonin syndrome.

7.3 Contraindications Women on Tamoxifen

Paroxetine and *fluoxetine* are to be *categorically avoided in tamoxifen users*. These SSRIs in particular are highly potent *inhibitors* of CYP2D6, the enzyme which converts tamoxifen to its most active metabolite endoxifen.

Safer choices, endorsed by NAMS, are the SSRI's escitalopram and citalopram and the SNRI's venlafaxine and desvenlafaxine.

7.4 Gabapentin (GABA)

Gabapentin is an anticonvulsant drug used to treat seizures in children and adults and is also FDA-approved for treating diabetic neuropathy and postherpetic neuralgia. Though FDA off label for this indication, many placebo-controlled trials have demonstrated GABA at 900 mg daily (300 mg TID) to reduce the frequency and intensity of VMS. One study actually showed that at the high dose of 2400 mg per day, GABA was in fact on par with the efficacy of conjugated equine estrogen (CEE 0.625 mg). However, its effectiveness was hindered by marked adverse effects of headache, dizziness, and disorientation [61, 63]. Its less threatening side effect also includes drowsiness; this agent may be an optimal choice for women whose VMS are associated with significant sleep disruption.

7.5 Clonidine

Clonidine, as mentioned previously, is a centrally acting alpha-2 adrenergic agonist that has been shown only slightly better efficacy to placebo [61, 64]. It was used rarely decades ago for treating VMS in patients with a contraindication or who simply declined estrogen. As it has both significantly more adverse effects (hypotension, lightheadedness, headache, dry mouth, sedation, dizziness, constipation, and significant rebound hypertension) as well as much less efficiency than SSRIs, SNRIs, and GABA, Clonidine is only mentioned for its historical significance.

8 Genitourinary Syndrome of Menopause

In 2014, the North American Menopause Society (NAMS) and the International Society for the Study of Women's Sexual Health (ISSWSH) convened to replace the term vulvo-vaginal atrophy (VVA) with a less socially stigmatizing and more descriptive term. Genito-urinary syndrome of menopause (GSM) became the new term for covering the full constellation of potential genital, urological, and sexual symptoms resulting from decreased estrogen and other sex steroid levels in menopause.

The most common symptoms may include, but are not limited to vaginal dryness, burning and irritation, painful sex that can evolve into secondary sexual dysfunction, bladder and urethral symptoms, recurrent vaginitis, more frequent and recurrent urinary tract infections (UTIs), urinary urgency, and dysuria. Untreated, the prevalence of this condition presenting with symptoms is 50% of all women in postmenopause.

Unlike VMS, GSM generally presents later in menopause, never resolves and gets worst over time if untreated. Abrupt or early menopause resulting from oophorectomy, chemotherapy, primary ovarian insufficiency, GNRH agonist therapy, or any other condition or treatment leading to sharp falls in estrogen will accelerate the rate of progression, severity of symptoms, level of sexual dysfunction, and general quality of life. GSM untreated affects all women over time in menopause to varying degrees and with especially bothersome symptoms in close to 50% of women in the United States [65].

In the VIVA survey of 3520 postmenopausal women aged 55–65 in the United Kingdom, the United States, Canada, and Scandinavian countries, 45% reported GSM symptoms and 75% endorsed a negative impact on quality of life. Only 4% of those reporting symptoms understood the cause and, of those who did, only 37% understood it was a chronic condition. Lastly, close to half queried (46%) were unaware of local estrogen and other treatment options [66]. In another more widely ranging survey of 2160 women aged 45–75, more than 90% endorsed symptoms of GSM and their symptom severity ran in tandem with quality of life severity [67].

Despite their negative impact on QOL, women will not seek help out of embarrassment or the belief that "this is part of natural aging" [67]. Sadly, breast cancer survivors often feel so grateful to be alive that they choose not to complain. As such, symptoms are not voluntarily endorsed, providers don't ask and the survivor suffers in silence. Worst, those who bravely endorse their GSM symptoms in breast cancer survivorship clinics will have them addressed less than 40% of the time by healthcare professionals [68].

9 Treatment Options

1. **Moisturizers and lubricants**

   Recommended as first line, women with sexually symptomatic GSM may try nonhormonal vaginal lubricants to be used during sex, vaginal moisturizers used several times a week as well as regular sexual activity. For severe GSM presenting with vaginal constriction and vaginismus, lubricated serially graduated vaginal dilators as well as pelvic floor therapy may be of benefit [69].
2. **Estrogen**

   GSM is one of four conditions for which estrogen is FDA approved and remains the "gold standard" treatment option. Low dose vaginal estrogen, arbitrarily defined as the 7.5 μg vaginal ring or the 10 μg tablet, results in minimal systemic absorption of (symbol less than or equal to) 20 pg/mL; this is well within the normal serum estradiol range of 0–30 pg/mL for postmenopausal women [70]. For women who concurrently suffer from both VMS and GSM, systemic estrogen (oral or transdermal with or without progestogen) usually suffices to treat both conditions. However, 10–15% of women with moderate to severe VMS will have such severe GSM that they will require both local vaginal estrogen as well as systemic estrogen [71]. Unlike systemic estrogen, a progestogen is not required with low-dose vaginal estrogen.
3. **Ospemiphene**

   Ospemiphene is an oral selective estrogen receptor modulator (SERM) that is FDA approved for the treatment of moderate dyspareunia as a result of GSM. An additional benefit is favorable effects on bone similar to raloxifene [1, 72], as well as no endometrial hyperplasia risk (with no progestogen needed). Disadvantages are that it may actually increase vasomotor symptoms (VMS) and the possible risk of venous thromboembolism (VTE).
4. **DHEA**

   Vaginal DHEA (Prasterone), for the treatment of GSM, is the brainchild of the late Professor Fernand Labrie (1937–2019) who pioneered the science of intracrinolgy and brilliantly created a product that epitomizes translational medicine. Intravaginal 6.5 mg dehydroepiandosterone (DHEA) ovule (Prasterone or Intrarosa) is FDA-approved in postmenopausal women with moderate-severe dyspareunia from GSM. A 12-week randomized placebo-controlled phase III clinical trial of intravaginal DHEA demonstrated marked improvement compared to placebo: by 12 weeks, parabasal cells decreased by 28%, superficial cells increased 8%, and vaginal pH decreased by 0.66 pH units over placebo. Dyspareunia decreased by 1.42 severity score units over placebo score unites ($P = 0.0002$) over placebo. On gynecological examination, vaginal secretions, epithelial integrity, epithelial surface thickness, and color all improved by 86–121% over placebo. Lastly, serum steroid levels, namely DHEA and its main metabolites (DHEA-S, testosterone, DHT, 4-dione, 5-diol, estrone, estradiol), remained well within normal postmenopausal values [73].

The mechanism of action of vaginal DHEA is based on the science of *intracrinology* whose discovery and elucidation is less than 30-years old and arguably more mechanistically complex than the classical mechanisms of *endocrinology*. According to mechanisms of endocrinology, a hormone such as estrogen is produced by its parent organ the ovary and released into the bloodstream and distributed quite randomly and indiscriminately to all body tissues and organs, leaving the tissue and organ specificity to the presence or absence in each cell of various levels and subtypes of hormone (e.g., estrogen) receptors. According to the mechanisms of intracrinology, there are over 30 steroid-forming enzymes specific for each peripheral tissue *within the cell* whose role is to convert a hormone present in that cell into another type of hormone (or hormones) strictly for intracellular and local action [74].

In the case of DHEA, the vaginal tissue-specific enzymes will transform DHEA into small amounts of both estrogen and testosterone for a uniquely and strictly intracellular and local action [74]. Additionally, humans and primates uniquely possess intracellular steroid inactivating enzymes—glucuronyl transferases and sulfotransferases—which inactivate estrogens and androgens at their local intracellular site of formation, hence cleverly preventing release into the bloodstream of biologically significant amounts of estradiol and testosterone [74]. Studies using highly sensitive assays show a very slight but statistically significant increase in serum estradiol and testosterone yet still falling in the lower half of normal postmenopausal values [75, 76]. As the product is relatively new, it has not yet been studied in breast cancer survivors nor have there yet been head-to-head trials with vaginal estrogen comparing serum hormone levels and efficacy. Nonetheless, vaginal DHEA is a novel invention that epitomizes the power and elegance of translational medicine.

10 Off-Label Options

10.1 Vaginal Testosterone

The off-label use of vaginal testosterone is only mentioned for completeness, but one should underscore it as controversial. Those in favor, quote the known fact that genitourinary tissues robustly express both estrogen as well as testosterone receptors [77]. As testosterone is converted to estradiol by the aromatase enzyme, it was posited that perhaps breast cancer survivors with GSM taking aromatase inhibitors (AIs) would be ideal candidates for vaginal testosterone as their AIs would prevent increased potentially risky serum estradiol levels. In a clinical trial on breast cancer survivors on AIs taking vaginal testosterone for GSM, the hypothesis was proven wrong with 12% having persistently elevated estradiol levels [78]. As there are no currently FDA-approved testosterone formulations (both local as well as systemic) for women, this limits its use to less tested compounded options. As there remain many other available options, one finds fewer reasons to advocate its use.

10.2 Vaginal Laser

The FDA has approved laser therapy for several medical indications including cosmetic dermatology, refractive eye surgery, dentistry, and general surgery (tumor removal, breast surgery, plastic surgery, and cataract removal) (FDA.gov website section on medical lasers).

There have been over 40 peer-reviewed clinical studies showing efficacy and safety in treating GSM in postmenopausal women as well as in breast cancer survivors with the micro-ablative fractional CO_2 laser. The mechanism of action, validated with pre and post-treatment pathology studies, is the stimulation of growth of new mature superficial vaginal epithelium replete with restored glycogen, neovascularization, and restored collagen and elastin. The laser energy's putative action is though the initiation of a "heat shock response" within the vaginal lamina propria which expresses heat shock protein #70 and other cofactors which in turn activate fibroblast precursors to fully mature and produce collagen. Electron microscopy elegantly performed by Salvatore et al. [79] demonstrates pretreatment endoplasmic reticulum with empty crypts that then fill with collagen fibrils after laser stimulation (Fig. 2).

Pathology studies pre and post-treatment demonstrate the lush re-epithelialization of vaginal mucosa replete with Hematoxylin and Eosin stained glycogen. The atrophic postmenopausal vaginal epithelium is restored to premenopausal health with the return of protective lactobacilli and, similar to the effects of vaginal estrogen, dyspareunia as well as other GSM symptoms such as recurrent vaginitis and UTIs improve [79] (Fig. 3).

The treatment is one option for breast cancer survivors who often have the most extreme GSM symptoms. In a retrospective study of 82 breast cancer survivors with GSM symptoms that failed nonestrogenic vaginal therapy who were given three treatments of vaginal CO2 laser over 4 months, showed quite significant improvements in dyspareunia and vaginal itching, dryness, burning, dysuria, and bleeding [80].

In comparing efficacy of vaginal estrogen to laser, the lack of randomized trials has been the major critique; one such study, the VeLVET, has just been completed and awaits publication.

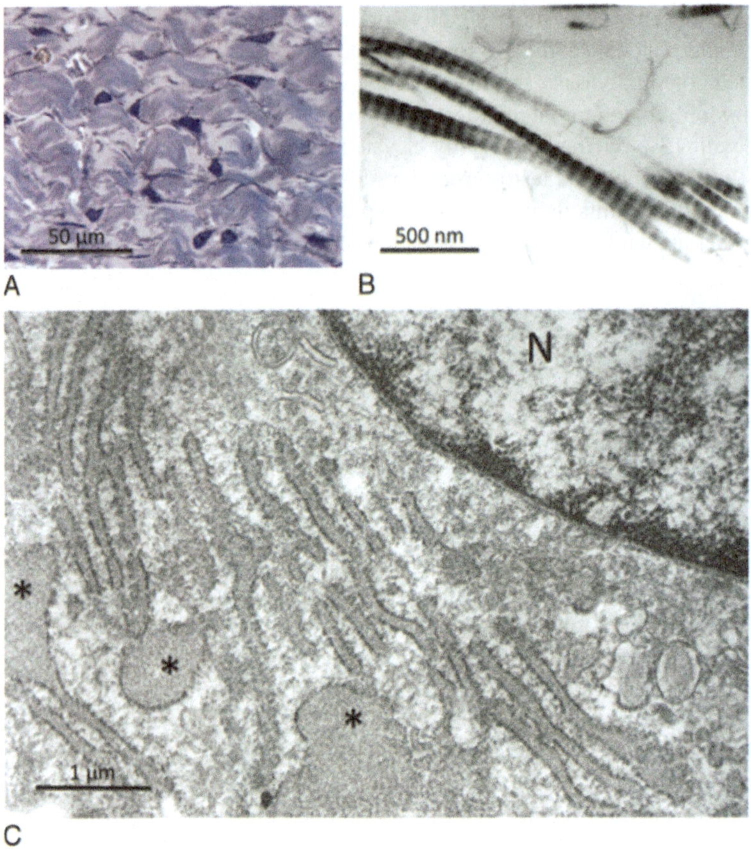

Fig. 2 (**a**) Fibroblasts surrounded by the extracellular matrix: compact bundles of collagen fibers are well distinguishable from the ground matrix (light microscopy, toluidine blue staining). (**b**) High-magnification electron microscopy of collagen microfibrils with characteristic banding, in close relationship with very thin filaments representing molecular components in the course of aggregation to form mature microfibrils (fibrillogenesis). (**c**) Part of a fibroblast under an electron microscope. The cytoplasm is filled with profiles of the rough endoplasmic reticulum, constituted by flattened cisternae transversally sectioned with a lot of ribosomes attached to membranes, and dilated vesicles continuous with membranes of the rough endoplasmic reticulum. Both these structures are filled with a finely filamentous material representing molecular precursors of collagen fibers. *N* nucleus. *Dilated vesicles

Vaginal Erbium YAG lasers (VEL), despite a shorter track record with fewer studies compared to microablative fractional CO2, hold similar promise and are currently under expanded trials. Data show that both energy systems have the enormous potential to resolve severe GSM symptoms and impaired quality of life in breast cancer survivors without the need for local hormone therapy.

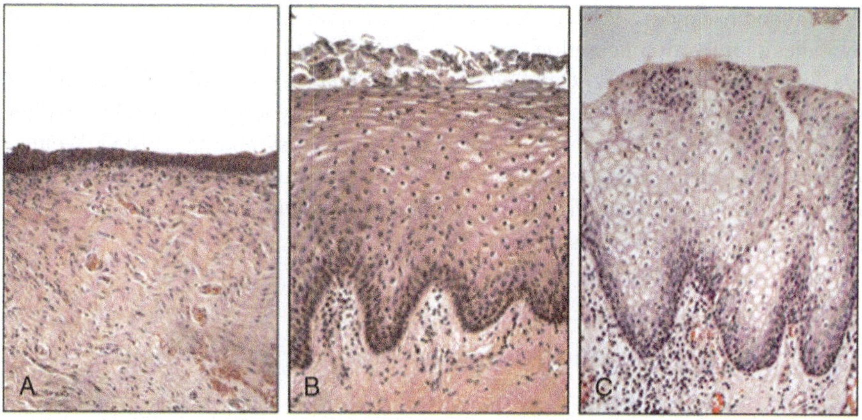

Fig. 3 Morphological findings from clinical practice. (**a**) Atrophic vaginal mucosa before fractional CO_2 laser treatment. (**b**) Vaginal mucosa of the same person 2 months after treatment. Note the lamina propria newly formed connective tissue with vessel-rich papillae, the thick stratified squamous epithelium, and normally shedding superficial cells. (**c**) Normal vaginal mucosa of a fertile-age woman (reported for comparison)

11 Osteoporosis Prevention

The third FDA-approved indication for postmenopausal estrogen use is for the *prevention* of osteoporosis but *not* the *treatment* of osteoporosis.

Osteoporosis is the most common cause of morbidity for women after the menopause transition (menopause practice) [1]. Osteoporotic hip fractures occur at a median age of 82 which leads to death within a year in 25%, long-term care needed in another 25%, and the remainder will have long-term loss of mobility [1]. Women have their peak bone mass at the age of 30, after which bone loss begins and finally accelerates at menopause with the loss of ovarian estrogen.

Estrogen is the most physiologic agent available to maintain bone mass to prevent osteoporosis. Standard dose estrogen, with or without a progestogen, has been thought to prevent bone loss in postmenopausal women by primarily inhibiting osteoclast-driven bone resorption and reducing the overall rate of bone remodeling (NAMS 2017 position statement) More recently, the estrogen-mediated orchestration of bone remodeling has been found to be much more complex with details still unfolding. Estrogen seems to have direct pleiotropic effects on osteoclasts, osteoblasts, and osteocytes resulting in decreased bone resorption, maintenance of bone formation, and inhibition of bone remodeling, respectively [84].

Whatever the details of estrogen's complex pleiotropic effects on bone finally demonstrate in the lab, standard dose MHT has been clinically proven to reduce all categories of osteoporotic fractures—namely hip, spine and non-spinal fractures in both observational as well as RCT's [3].

Estrogen has a dose-related effect on bone mineral density, and bone protection dwindles rapidly after cessation. An ideal clinical case for the use of MHT for the prevention of osteoporosis would be in a woman who has no medical contraindications to estrogen, is in the "early window" (i.e., age younger than 60 or within 10 years of menopause onset), and also has vasomotor symptoms (VMS). Women with premature menopause, without contraindications, are better served with estrogen than with a bone-specific treatment which have their potential adverse effects and whose duration of use is limited [3].

12 Primary Ovarian Insufficiency and Early Menopause

Primary ovarian insufficiency (POI), the currently preferred term to replace primary ovarian failure and premature menopause, is defined as menopause before the age of 40 diagnosed by at least 4 months of amenorrhea and 2 menopausal FSH levels 1 month apart. The etiology is vast, ranging from iatrogenic (cancer treatments—oophorectomy, chemotherapy, radiation), genetic (fragile-X syndrome, Turner syndrome), autoimmune (adrenal, thyroid), infectious, or environmental. Yet the cause remains unknown in 90% of cases [86]. Early menopause occurs in women with the above findings who are older than 40 but younger than 45.

Both conditions, especially POI, have many health risks directly related to ovarian hormone deficiency, primarily estrogen [3, 87]. Unlike women in natural menopause, these younger women should be viewed as having a *pathologic* state of estrogen deficiency compared with their age-related peers with normal ovarian function, and in these scenarios the term "Hormone Replacement Therapy" (as opposed to Menopausal Hormone Therapy) is actually more appropriate [87].

Adverse health effects include persistent and severe menopausal symptoms of both VMS (hot flashes, night sweats, insomnia) and GSM (vaginal dryness, dyspareunia, decreased sexual desire, vaginitis, urinary frequency, dysuria, recurrent UTIs), decreased bone density and increased risk of fracture, infertility, increased risk of mood disorders such as depression and anxiety, increased risk of cognitive decline, dementia and Parkinson's disease, sexual dysfunction, increased risk of thyroid and adrenal autoimmune disease, increased risk of prediabetes and type 2 diabetes, dry eye syndrome, increased risk of cardiovascular disease, and overall increased mortality risk.

Sadly, over 50% of women with POI either refuse to take HRT, start it many years after the diagnosis, or discontinue before age 45. As such, difference between *replacement* therapy and *extension* therapy should be clearly explained to patients; namely that they are missing a hormone whose absence is negatively impacting the long list of adverse health effects and whose replacement would mitigate them to restore health and quality of life.

There is universal consensus from the North American Menopause Society (NAMS), the American Society for Reproductive Medicine (ASRM), the European

Society of Human Reproduction and Embryology (ESHRE), The Endocrine Society (ES), the International Menopause Society (IMS), and the European Menopause and Andropause Society (EMAS) that in women with premature ovarian insufficiency (POI), systemic MHT, without contraindications, is recommended *at least* until the age of natural menopause. POI is also the fourth FDA-approved indication for MHT.

Yet, there remains no consensus for dosage, formulation, and route of administration of estrogen and progestogen for POI as for all other indications. Sullivan, Sarrell, and Nelson [87] address the question for POI with a thought experiment: the ultimate lofty design of an artificial ovary that would deliver a constant parenteral flow of the correct mix of hormones to mimic endogenous ovarian production throughout a menstrual cycle. The first crude baby step in this direction would be a transdermal patch that delivers 0.100 mg of estradiol per day. This would supply the average serum estradiol levels of 100 pg/mL that women with normal ovarian function are exposed to over the full menstrual cycle. The transdermal route of estrogen is preferred over oral as the risk of venous thromboembolism (VTE), as well as stroke is markedly reduced by avoiding complications resulting from the oral route's first-pass effect on the liver. In the large Estrogen and Thromboembolism Risk (ESTHER) study performed on postmenopausal women, the odds ratio for venous thromboembolism for women using oral estrogen was 4.2 compared with 0.9 for transdermal users [87, 88]. Although micronized progesterone (natural or body-identical) has fewer risks and more benefits than the synthetic progestins such as medroxy-progesterone acetate (MPA) and as such are currently in favor over the latter used in the WHI, there is lack of consensus on which progestogen is best for treating women with POI who have a uterus. The NIH performed a 3-year study [87, 89] looking at the effect of full replacement dosing on bone mineral density on women with POI with transdermal estradiol 100 μg/mL daily with oral medroxy-progesterone acetate (10 mg per day for 12 days per month). Bone mineral density improved by as much as 8% at the femoral neck over 3 years as opposed to healthy age-matched controls who lost bone density untreated. The addition of transdermal testosterone to the HRT regimen did not provide additional bone density. The investigators chose MPA as their progestin over micronized progesterone due to lack of endometrial protection data with the latter at such high (full replacement) doses of estradiol. The PEPI group only examined and documented oral micronized progesterone's ability to induce endometrial secretory changes with lower postmenopausal estrogen dosing and not the higher HRT dose used for POI patients.

Transdermal estradiol in higher doses with adequate endometrial protection with a progestogen seems to have better maintenance of bone mineral density compared with oral contraceptives [3, 27, 90, 91]. Furthermore, oral contraceptives were developed to suppress ovulation in normally cycling women and, as such, supply supraphysiologic levels that provide no additional benefit beyond that of HRT with much added risk, namely increased risk of thromboembolism, stroke, increased blood pressure, unfavorable lipid profiles, and general increased cardiometabolic risk [87].

The only consideration for use of oral contraceptive with a patch during the placebo week over HRT would be for psychological benefit in younger women [3].

The psychological impact resulting from the caretaker's delivery of the diagnosis of POI cannot be underscored enough. POI has been associated with poor psychosocial functioning, higher levels of depression and anxiety, low self-esteem, higher perceived stress, and lower sexual well-being [92]. Younger women, particularly those in their late 20s will be more devastated by the diagnosis carrying loss of fertility and will generally be able to cope less well with any experienced menopausal symptoms and as such would benefit from a peer-based support network. All women should be informed sensitively and in an unrushed manner to be able to ask questions and should be given timely follow-up appointment and connected with informational and support networks.

13 Vasomotor Symptoms and Cardiovascular Disease Risk

Only recently, a compelling yet enigmatic body of data has emerged linking vasomotor symptoms (VMS) with preclinical markers of cardiovascular disease.

From the large SWAN study that delineated the previously noted four types of trajectories/patterns of VMS (i.e., early onset VMS, consistently high VMS [the Super Flashers]), late onset VMS, and persistently low VMS), a subgroup of 811 women were examined to look at the association between individual VMS pattern and carotid artery disease risk.[1] Enrollees were healthy white, black, Hispanic, and Chinese women aged 42–52 with a uterus and ovaries, not on OCP/MHT, 1–2 menses in past 3 months, and no history of stroke or prior MI. They were seen annually for completed measures of VMS, bloodwork, and physical measures for 13 years: a carotid artery ultrasound was performed at the final annual study visit. The results showed that the women with the pattern of early onset VMS as well as those with persistently high VMS had higher carotid artery intima media thickness (CIMT) compared with those with persistently low VMS. Notably, when adjusting for covariables such as race/ethnicity and blood pressure, only the early onset VMS group had higher CIMT compared with the persistently low VMS group [45, 93].

The WISE (Women's Ischemia Syndrome Evaluation) study was a prospective study of 936 patients who initially underwent clinically indicated (to further evaluate signs and symptoms suspect for an ischemic event) coronary angiography and then followed annually for fatal and nonfatal CVD events for a total median of 9.3 years. Thurston et al. [114] performed a substudy of 104 women who were all postmenopausal, over 50, and not taking hormone therapy (HT)

[1] Carotid ultrasound measurement of carotid artery intimal media thickness (CIMT), also used in the KRONOS and KEEPS studies to test the timing hypothesis, is an accepted surrogate for measurement of CVD risk.

examining the association between endothelial dysfunction and VMS patterns. Ultrasound of the brachial artery was used to test for reduced flow-mediated dilation (FMD).[2] Women with early onset VMS—notably before age 42—had lower FMD, hence poorer endothelial function, than either the women who never had VMS or those with later onset VMS. In addition, women with early onset VMS had the highest CVD mortality and in fact, when adjusted for multiple covariate CVD risk factors (such as hypertension, BMI, diabetes, ever smoker, dyslipidemia, former HT use), the CVD mortality risk actually became stronger (i.e. unadjusted CVD mortality hazard ratio (HR) of 2.34 increased to 2.83 when adjusted for covariate CVD risk factors.

These prior studies were limited by VMS data being subjective recollection which can both fragment over time and be influenced by negative mood, itself being related to both CVD risk and VMS.

As such, Thurston et al. [115] prospectively studied 300 nonsmoking healthy unmedicated women aged 40–60 with objective physiological recording of VMS (in tandem with subjective diary VMS collections) and looked at their hematologic CVD risk factors and carotid artery status. Even though they had somewhat favorable CVD risk factor profiles, almost half of the participants had carotid plaque. Among those reporting VMS, the frequency of VMS (both diary-collected and physiologically recorded) was associated with higher carotid IMT as well as more plaque in a dose–response relation. Even after controlling for CVD risk factors, the association between VMS frequency and increased coronary IMT remained robust [115].

The mechanism linking VMS to CVD risk remains enigmatic. As it awaits deciphering, this compelling link should be a loud wake-up call for clinicians and investigators alike to broaden the timeframe for screening women for cardiovascular disease; specifically, to not only use menopause as the "sentinel event" for screening for preclinical CVD risk factors but to perhaps consider screening those with persistent and severe VMS even earlier in the menopause transition [108-113, 116, 117].

14 Other Benefits of MHT

14.1 Joints and Muscles

Estrogen's beneficial effect on general joint health with the symptomatic improvement of arthritis and arthralgia is supported by many studies though the mechanism is unclear [3]. When combined with exercise, estrogen seems to help maintain

[2] FMD is performed by first measuring the resting diameter of the brachial artery with ultrasound, then distally placing a blood pressure cuff and stressing the artery by inflating it 40 mm above the systolic BP for 4 min, then deflating the cuff and, 2 min later, measuring the final brachial artery diameter. The calculation formula is FMD = 100 × peak diameter after cuff deflation minus resting diameter divided by resting diameter) is an accepted surrogate marker for endothelial dysfunction.

muscle mass and strength and thus attenuate sarcopenia. The potential health benefits include reduced sarcopenia, while frailty is linked to falls, hip fractures, and increased mortality. Skeletal muscle expresses estrogen receptors as the joint tissue; beyond that, the mechanism by which estrogen works on muscle mass is still enigmatic [3].

14.2 Metabolism

Contrary to popular lay belief, MHT is not associated with weight gain. In fact, it is menopause and its hormone changes that are associated with increased android/abdominal fat accumulation (IMS pos). Conversely, MHT reduces overall fat mass, improves insulin sensitivity, and significantly reduces the number of cases of new-onset type 2 diabetes mellitus (DM) [3]. The benefits are seen in both E alone as well as E/P but more robust with E/P reducing type 2 DM incidence by as much as 40%; unfortunately, the benefit vanishes when MHT is stopped. Diabetes prevention with MHT as a sole indication is currently not endorsed by the FDA or any menopause societies, but is a powerful secondary benefit of MHT. The primary recommendation for diabetes prevention in prediabetics remains caloric restriction and exercise with the goal of losing 7% of body weight.

14.3 Colorectal Cancer

The bulk of observational studies show that users of oral MHT have a lower incidence of colorectal cancer. The initial results of the WHI in all age categories reported a 38% lower risk specifically in the E/P arm compared with placebo while on treatment. However, later postintervention results showed no lowering of risk of colorectal cancer with either E/P or E alone. It seems as though the putative risk reduction with colorectal cancer while on therapy vanishes once therapy is stopped just as with bone health, metabolic health, and urogenital health.

15 Risks

15.1 Venous Thromboembolism (VTE), Gallbladder Disease, Stroke

The risks of venous thromboembolism, gallbladder disease, and stroke are small, particularly without risk factors such as obesity, thrombophilia, or prior history of the above. They are associated with oral estrogen though its hepatic "first pass" effect. The use of transdermal estrogen instead or oral significantly reduces these risks [94].

15.2 Breast Cancer

Cardiovascular disease (CVD) is the leading cause of death in men as well as women. In women, 1 in 3.3 deaths are attributable to CVD compared to 1 in 32 attributable to breast cancer. Yet women are far more fearful of the latter which often deters their use of MHT. Does HRT, in a low-risk patient, indeed increase the risk of invasive breast cancer? And by how much compared with other modifiable known risk factors?

Most studies, including the WHI, indicate a small increased risk of invasive breast cancer with E/P—but in these studies, the P is always a progestin (synthetic progestogen such as MPA used in the WHI) [91]. Micronized progesterone (MP) and the synthetic progestins have markedly different effects on breast tissue [91]. Progestogens are a highly heterogeneous group lacking a "class effect": they differ in their chemical structure, metabolism, pharmacokinetics, affinity to progesterone receptors (PR), and, perhaps most importantly, highly variable relative binding affinities to other steroid receptors, androgen receptors (AR), mineralocorticoid receptors (MR), and glucocorticoid receptors (GR); as such, their biological and clinical effects are enormously varied [90].

A germane example is that micronized progesterone, the natural progesterone, is highly selective to progesterone receptors yet lacks glucocorticoid activity; conversely, MPA not only binds to the PR with even greater affinity than natural progesterone but also binds to the glucocorticoid receptor (GR) with even greater affinity than native cortisol [90].

Recent data suggest that micronized progesterones, unlike synthetic progestogens, do not appear to increase the risk of breast cancer [91, 95, 96]. In the French E3N cohort study of 80,377 postmenopausal women followed for over 8 years, users of estrogens with micronized progesterone did not have an increased risk over never users (RR 1.00; 95% CI 0.83–1.22). In contrast, both users of estrogen only as well as users of estrogens with progestins (synthetic progestogens) had increased risks over the never users (RR 1.29 and RR 1.69, respectively) [91, 95].

In addition, current thinking is that MHT has a promoter effect rather than an initiating effect on breast cancer [91, 97]. Santen [97] reviewed a mathematical model which proposes 16 years to be the average time it takes for a single breast cancer cell to grow to a clinically detectable lesion. The basis for the model is average doubling time of 200 days and the need for 30 doublings to reach a mammographically detectable threshold size of 1.1 cm. As such, the vast majority (94%) of the tumors diagnosed over the 7-year duration of the WHI E/P were occult tumors already in situ at the time the study began. Moreover, the promoting effect of a more hazardous regimen no longer favored (i.e., CEE/MPA vs. estradiol/micronized progesterone) has a HR of 1.26 which is higher than that of drinking one glass of wine and less than two glasses of wine daily [98, 99].

15.3 *MHT for Primary Prevention of CVD and Other Chronic Diseases*

With the exception of the prevention of osteoporosis, neither the FDA nor any of the menopause societies endorse the use of MHT in women who do not have the indications of bothersome VMS, GSM, or POI—for primary prevention of CVD and other chronic disease. The U.S. Preventive Services Task Force (USPSTF) issued a Draft Recommendation in 2017 condemning the use of MHT for primary prevention with a D recommendation [100]. A group of leading pundits in the menopausal orbit penned a compelling and elegant rebuttal to the USPSTF's erroneous statement. Some highlights of the paper are as follows: "considering the relative importance of coronary heart disease, fragility fractures, colorectal cancer and diabetes to the public health—alongside potential harms—the balance is clearly toward benefit from MHT when initiated within 10 years of menopause in women with appropriate indications, with continuation thereafter for an indeterminate period for the prevention of chronic diseases" [101]. This view, they highlight, is shared in both the International Menopause Society's (IMS) latest position statement as well as by the North American Menopause Society's (NAMS) latest position statement [3] (in turn endorsed by 35 national and international medical societies) [118].

As coronary heart disease is the leading cause of death in women, they compare the strengths of available primary prevention strategies. Lifestyle interventions, often with low compliance, will reduce the 10-year coronary risk by a maximum of 12–14%. Although statins and aspirin are used for prevention in men, they argue that there is little statistically valid data supporting their use in women for primary prevention of CHD or reduced mortality [81, 102–107]. In addition, they argue that statin therapy—advocated by the USPSTF in place of MHT for primary prevention of CHD—may increase the risk of diabetes in women [82], while MHT is protective. By contrast, Mikolla et al. [83] demonstrated in another study of close to 500,000 Finnish women on estradiol-based MHT that users compared to age-matched nonusers had decreased risks of CHD death by 18–54%. Moreover, the risk reduction was highest in those with the longest duration of use of MHT. In addition, risk of stroke death as well as all-cause mortality was reduced.

16 Summary and Conclusions

Menopausal hormone therapy offered to postmenopausal women without contraindications appears to be the most effective treatment for vasomotor symptoms, genitourinary syndrome of menopause, prevention of osteoporosis, and for both symptom relief as well as chronic disease prevention and reduction in all-cause mortality in women with primary ovarian insufficiency, premature menopause, or iatrogenic menopause. In addition to treating symptoms and improving quality of life, menopausal hormone therapy arguably appears to be the most effective modality for primary prevention of cardiovascular disease as well as prevention of other chronic illnesses such as osteoporosis, colorectal cancer, diabetes, metabolic syndrome, and possibly dementia.

When abiding by the rules of the timing hypothesis namely if *starting* before the age of 60 or within 10 years of the onset of menopause, in women without contraindications, the highlighted benefits seem to outweigh the risks. The menopause transition should be targeted as a sentinel event to screen for preclinical markers for future cardiometabolic disease. The newly discovered "high risk" cohort of women with early onset and/or severe vasomotor symptoms deserves particular scrutiny as they have a greater risk for preclinical cardiovascular and possibly other chronic diseases.

The timing hypothesis and its body of evidence has radically changed our views post-WHI and in turn has radically changed our essential clinical practice principles. For almost 10 years post-WHI, the consensus for treating all postmenopausal symptomatic women without contraindications was to "give the lowest dose for the shortest amount of time." The current consensus is that HT should be "individualized to identify the most appropriate HT type, dose, formulation, route of administration, timing of initiation and duration of use, using the best available evidence to maximize benefits and minimize risks, and periodic re-evaluation of the benefits and risks of continuing or discontinuing HT" [3].

Unfortunately, the lay community, as well as many of our own esteemed medical colleagues of other specialties are too often unaware of this paradigm shift and instead remain in post-WHI darkness. Until everyone is properly educated, women's health may arguably suffer.

References

1. Menopause practice: a clinician's guide. North American Menopause Society; 2014.
2. Murphy SL, Xu J, Kockanek KD. Deaths: final data for 2010. Natl Vital Stat Rep. 2013;61(4):1–117.
3. Pinkerton JV, Aguirre FS, Blake J, Hodis H, et al. The 2017 hormone therapy position statement of the North American Menopause Society. Menopause. 24(7):728–53.
4. Stuenkel C, Davis SR, Gompel A, et al. Treatment of symptoms of the menopause: an Endocrine Society Clinical Practice guideline. J Clin Endocrinol Metab. 2015;100:3975–4011.
5. Sayegh R, Awwad JT. Five decades of hormone therapy research: the long, the short, and the inconclusive. In: Essentials of menopause management. Springer; 2017.
6. Bush TL, et al. Estrogen use and all cause mortality: preliminary results from the lipid research clinics program follow-up study. JAMA. 1983;249:903–6.
7. Ross RK, et al. Menopausal oestrogen therapy and protection from death from ischemic heart disease. Lancet. 1981;1:858–60.
8. Pfeffer RI, et al. Coronary risk and estrogen use in postmenopausal women. Am. J Epidemiol. 1978;107:479–87.
9. Bain C, et al. Use of postmenopausal hormones and risk of myocardial infarction. Circulation. 1981;64:42–6.

10. Lobo RA, Pickar JH, Stevenson JC, Mack WJ, Hodis HN. Back to the future: hormone replacement therapy as part of a prevention strategy for women at the onset of menopause. Atherosclerosis. 2016;254:296–304.
11. Stampfer MJ, et al. Estrogen replacement therapy and coronary heart disease: a quantitative assessment of the epidemiologic evidence. Prev Med. 1991;20:47–63.
12. Grodstein F, et al. Postmenopausal hormone therapy and mortality. N Engl J Med. 1997;336:1769–75.
13. Yaffe K, et al. Estrogen therapy in postmenopausal women: effects on cognitive function and dementia. JAMA. 1998;279:688–95.
14. Henderson BE, et al. Decreased mortality in users of estrogen replacement therapy. Arch Intern Med. 1991;151:75–8.
15. Grady D, et al. Hormone therapy to prevent disease and prolong life in postmenopausal women. Ann Intern Med. 1992;117:1016–37.
16. Stampfer MJ, et al. A prospective study of postmenopausal estrogen therapy and coronary heart disease. N Engl J Med. 1985;313:1044–9.
17. Bush TL, et al. Cardiovascular mortality and noncontraceptive use of estrogen in women: results from the lipid research clinics follow-up study. Circulation. 1987;75:1102–9.
18. Henderson BE, Paganini-Hill A, Ross RK. Estrogen replacement therapy and protection from acute myocardial infarction. Am J Obstet Gynecol. 1988;159:312–7.
19. American College of Physicians. Guidelines for counselling postmenopausal women about preventive hormone therapy. Ann Intern Med. 1992;117:1038–41.
20. Greendale GA. Symptom relief and side effects of postmenopausal hormones: results from the PEPI trial Obstet. Gynecologie. 1998;92:982–8.
21. Writing Group for the PEPI trial. Effects of hormone therapy on bone mineral density: results from the PEPI tria. JAMA. 1996;276:1389–96.
22. Hully S. Randomized trial of estrogen plus progestin for secondary prevention of coronary heart disease in postmenopausal women. JAMA. 1998;280:605.
23. Miller V, Clarkson T. Women, hormones and clinical trials: a beginning, not an end. J Appl Physiol. 2005;99:381.
24. Langer RD. The evidence base for HRT: what can we believe. Climacteric. 2017;20:91–6.
25. Lobo R. Hormone-replacement therapy: current thinking. Nat Rev Endocrinol. 2017; 13:220.
26. Sprague BL, et al. Sustained decline in postmenopausal use: results from the National Health and Nutrition Examination Survey. Obstet Gynecol. 2012;120:595–603.
27. Karim R, et al. Hip fracture in postmenopausal women after cessation of hormone therapy: results from a prospective study from a large HMO. Menopause. 2011;18:1172–7.
28. Islam S, et al. Trend in incidence of osteoporosis-related fractures among 40-69 year-old women: analysis of claims database, 2000-2005. Menopause. 2009;16:77–83.
29. Mikkola TS, Tuomikowski P, Lyytinen H, et al. Increased cardiovascular mortality risk in women discontinuing postmenopausal hormone therapy. J Clin Endocrinol Metab. 2015;100(12):4588–94.
30. Sarrel P, et al. The mortality toll of estrogen avoidance: an analysis of excess deaths among hysterectomized women aged 50-59 years. Am J Public Health. 2013;103:1583–8.
31. Lacroix AZ, Chlebowski RT, Manson JE, et al. Health outcomes after stopping conjugated equine estrogens among postmenopausal women with prior hysterectomy: a randomized controlled trial. JAMA. 2011;305:1305–14.
32. Burger HG, et al. Evidence-based assessment of the impact of the WHI on women's health. Climacteric. 2012;15:281–7.
33. Marko K, Simon JA. Clinical trials in menopause. Menopause. 2018;25:217.
34. Rossouw JE, Prentice RL, Manson JE, et al. Postmenopausal hormone therapy and risk of cardiovascular disease by age and years since menopause. JAMA. 2007;297:1465–77.

35. Salpeter SR, Walsh JM, Grayber E, Salpeter EE. Brief report: coronary heart disease events associated with hormone therapy in younger and older women. A meta-analysis. J Gen Intern Med. 2006;21:363–6.
36. Clarkson TB, Mehaffey M. Coronary heart disease of females: lessons learned from nonhuman primates. Am J Primatol. 2009;71:785–93.
37. Clarkson TB, Melendez GC, Appt SE. Timing hypothesis for postmenopausal hormone therapy: its origin, current status, and future. Menopause. 2013;20(3):342–53.
38. Mendelsohn ME, Karas RH. Molecular and cellular basis of cardiovascular gender differences. Science. 2005;308:1583–7.
39. Harman SM, Black DM, Naftolin F, et al. Arterial imaging outcomes and cardiovascular risk factors in recently menopausal women: a randomized trial. Ann Intern Med. 2014;161:249–60.
40. Miller VM, Naftolin F, Asthana S, et al. The Kronos Early Estrogen Prevention Study (KEEPS): what have we learned? Menopause. 2019;26(9):1–14.
41. Taylor HS, Tal A, Pal L, et al. Effects of oral versus transdermal estrogen therapy on sexual function in early post-menopause: ancillary study of the Kronos Early Estrogen Prevention Study (KEEPS). JAMA Intern Med. 2017;177:1471–9.
42. Hodis HN, Mack WJ, Shoupe D, et al. Methods and baseline cardiovascular data from the early versus late intervention trial with estradiol testing the menopausal hormone timing hypothesis. Menopause. 2014;22(4):391–401.
43. Sriprasert I, Hodis HN, Karim R, Stancyk FZ, Shoupe D, Henderson VW, Mack W. Differential effect of plasma estradiol on subclinical atherosclerosis progression in early vs late postmenopause. J Clin Endocrinol Metab. 2019;104(2):2930300.
44. Sturdee DW, Hunter MS, Maki PM, et al. The menopausal hot flush: a review. Climacteric. 2017;20(4):296–305.
45. Thurston RC. Vasomotor symptoms: natural history, physiology, and links with cardiovascular health. Climacteric. 2018;21(2):96–100.
46. Smith RL, Gallicchio LM, Flaws JA. Understanding the complex relationships underlying hot flashes: a Bayesian network approach. Menopause. 2018;25(2):182–90.
47. Carson MY, Thurston RC. Childhood abuse and vasomotor symptoms among midlife women. Menopause. 2019;26(10):1–7.
48. Freedman RR. Menopausal hot flashes: mechanisms, endocrinology, treatment. J Steroid Biochem Mol Biol. 2014;142:115–20.
49. Rance NE, Dacks PA, Mittleman-Smith M, et al. Modulation of body temperature and LH secretion by hypothalamic KNDy (kisspeptin, neurokinin B, and dynorphin) neurons: a novel hypothesis on the mechanism of hot flushes. Front Neuroendocrinol. 2013;34:211–27.
50. Casper RF, Yen SSC. Menopausal flushes: effect of pituitary gonadotropin desensitization by a potent luteinizing hormone-releasing factor agonist. J Clin Endocrinol Metab. 1981;53:1056–8.
51. Gambone J, Meldrum DR, Laufer L, et al. Further delineation of hypothalamic dysfunction responsible for menopausal hot flashes. J Clin Endocrinol Metab. 1984;59:1097–102.
52. Szeliga A, Czyzk A, Podfigurna A, Genazzani AD, Meczelalski B. The role of kisspeptin/neurokinin B/dynorphin neurons in pathomechanism of vasomotor symptoms in postmenopausal women: from physiology to potential therapeutic applications. Gynecol Endocrinol. 2018;34(11):913–9.
53. Skorupskaite K, George J, Anderson R. The Kisspeptin-GNRH pathway in human reproductive health and disease. Hum Reprod Update. 2014;20(4):485–500.
54. Padilla S, Johnson C, Barker F, Patterson M, Palmiter R. A neural circuit underlying the generation of hot flushes. Cell Rep. 2018;24:271–7.
55. Prague J, Roberts R, Dhillo W. Neurokinin 3 receptor antagonism rapidly improves vasomotor symptoms with sustained duration of action. Menopause. 2018;25(8):862–9.

56. Crandall CJ, Manson J, Hohensee C, et al. Association of genetic variation in the tachykinin receptor 3 locus with hot flashes and night sweats in the Women's Health Initiative study. Menopause. 2017;24:252–61.
57. Prague JK, Roberts RE, Comninos AN, et al. Neurokinin 3 receptor antagonism as a novel treatment for menopausal hot flushes: a phase 2, randomised, double-blind, placebo-controlled trial. Lancet. 2017;389(10081):1809–20.
58. Maclennan AH, Broadbent JL, Lester S, Moore V. Oral oestrogen and combined oestrogen/progestogen therapy versus placebo for hot flushes. Cochrane Database System Rev. 2004;4:CD002978.
59. Ockene JK, Barad DH, Cochrane BB, et al. Symptom experience after discontinuing use of estrogen plus progestin. JAMA. 2005;294:183–93.
60. Brunner RL, Aragaki A, Barnabei V, et al. Menopausal symptom experience before and after stopping estrogen therapy in the Women's Health Initiative randomized, placebo-controlled trial. Menopause. 2010;17:946–54.
61. Carpenter J, Gass M, Maki PM. Nonhormonal management of menopause-associated vasomotor symptoms: 2015 position statement of the North American Menopause Society. Menopause. 2015;22(11):1155–74.
62. Simon JA, Portman DJ, Kaunitz AM, et al. Low-dose paroxetine 7.5 mg for menopausal VMS: two randomized controlled trials. Menopause. 2013;20:1027–35.
63. Reddy SY, Warner H, Guttoso T Jr, et al. Gabapentin, estrogen, and placebo for treating hot flushes: a randomized controlled trial. Obstet Gynecol. 2006;108:41–8.
64. Nelson HD, Vesco KK, Haney E, et al. Nonhormonal therapies for menopausal hot flashes: systematic review and meta-analysis. JAMA. 2006;295:2057–71.
65. Nappi RE, Palacios S, Particco M, Panay N. The REVIVE (real Women's views of treatment options for menopausal vaginal changes) survey in Europe: country-specific comparisons of postmenopausal women's perceptions, experiences, and needs. Maturitas. 2016;91:81–90.
66. Nappi RE, Kokot-Kierepa M. Vaginal Health: Insights, Views, and Attitudes (VIVA)—results from an international survey. Climacteric. 2012;15:36–44.
67. Nappi RE, Palacios S, Bruyniks N, et al. The burden of vulvovaginal atrophy on women's daily living: implications on quality of life from a face-to-face real-life survey. Menopause. 2019;26(5):485–91.
68. Cook E, Iglehart E, Baum G, et al. Missing documentation in breast cancer survivors: genitourinary syndrome of menopause. Menopause. 2017;24(12):1360–4.
69. Management of symptomatic vulvovaginal atrophy: 2013 position statement of The North American Menopause Society. Menopause. 2013;20(9):888–902.
70. Santen RJ. Vaginal administration of estradiol: effects of dose, preparation and timing on plasma estradiol levels. Climacteric. 2015;18:121–34.
71. Rahn DD, Carberry C, Sanses TV, et al. Vaginal estrogen for genitourinary syndrome of menopause: a systematic review. Obstet Gynecol. 2015;124:1147–56.
72. Soe LH, Wurz GT, Koa CJ, et al. Ospemiphene for the treatment of dyspareunia associated with vulvar and vaginal atrophy: potential benefits in bone and breast Int. J Women's Health. 2013;5:605–11.
73. Labrie F, Archer D, Koltun W, et al. Efficacy of intravaginal dehydroepiandrosterone (DHEA) on moderate to severe dyspareunia and vaginal dryness, symptoms of vulvovaginal atrophy, and the genitourinary syndrome of menopause. Menopause. 2016;25(11):1339–53.
74. Labrie F, Belanger A, Pellitier G, Martel C, Archer D, Utian W. Science of intracrinology in postmenopausal women. Menopause. 2017;24(6):702–12.
75. Faubion S, Stuenkel C, Chism L, Kaunitz AM, Parish SJ, Pinkerton JV, Shapiro M, Simon JA, Kingsberg SA. Management of genitourinary syndrome of menopause in women with or at high risk for breast cancer: consensus recommendations from the North American Menopause Society and the International Society for the Study of Women's Sexual Health. Menopause. 2018;25(6):596–608.

76. Martel C, Labrie F, Archer DF, et al. Serum steroid concentrations remain within normal postmenopausal values in women receiving daily 6.5 mg intravaginal prasterone for 12 weeks. J Steroid Biochem Mol Biol. 2016;159:142–53.
77. Hodgins M, Spike R, Mackie R, MacLean A. An immunohistochemical study of androgen, oestrogen, and progesterone receptors in the vulva and vagina. Br J Obstet Gynaecol. 1998;105:216–22.
78. Melisko M, Goldman M, Hwang J, et al. Vaginal testosterone cream vs estradiol vaginal ring for vaginal dryness or decreased libido in women receiving aromatase inhibitors for early-stage breast cancer: a randomized clinical trial. JAMA Oncol. 20171;3:313–9.
79. Salvatore S, Maggiore ULR, Athanasiou S, et al. Histological study on the effects of microablative fractional CO2 laser on atrophic vaginal tissue: an ex vivo study. Menopause. 2015;22(8):845–9.
80. Pagano T, De Rosa P, Vallone R, et al. Fractional micro-ablative CO2 laser in breast cancer survivors affected by iatrogenic vulvovaginal atrophy after failure of non-estrogenic treatments: a retrospective study. Menopause. 2018;25:657–62.
81. Ogawa H, Nakayama M, Morimoto T. Low-dose aspirin for primary prevention of atherosclerotic events in patients with type 2 diabetes: a randomized controlled trial. JAMA. 2008;300:2134–41.
82. Sattar N, Preiss D, Murray HM, et al. Statins and risk of incident diabetes: a collaborative meta-analysis of randomized statin trials. Lancet. 2010;375:725–42.
83. Mikkola TS, Tuomikoski P, Lyytinen H, et al. Estradiol-based post-menopausal hormone therapy and risk of cardiovascular and all-cause mortality. Menopause. 2015;22:976–83.
84. Khosla S, Oursler MJ, Monroe DG. Estrogen and the skeleton. Trends Endocrinol Metab. 2012;23(11):576–81.
85. Savolainen-Peltonen H, Tuomikoski P, Korhonen P, et al. Cardiac death risk in relation to the age at initiation or the progestin component of hormone therapies. J Clin Endocrin Metab. 2016;101:2794–801.
86. Nelson LM. Primary ovarian insufficiency. NEJM. 2009;360(6):606–14.
87. Sullivan SD, Sarrel PM, Nelson LM. Hormone replacement therapy in young women with primary ovarian insufficiency and early menopause. Fertil Steril. 2016;106(7):1588–99.
88. Scarabin PY, Oger E, Plu-Bureau G. Differential association of oral and transdermal oestrogen-replacement therapy with venous thromboembolism risk. Lancet. 2003;362:428–32.
89. Popat VB, Calis KA, Kalantaridou SN, et al. Bone mineral density in young women with primary ovarian insufficiency: results of a three-year randomized controlled trial of physiological transdermal estradiol and testosterone replacement. J Clin Endocrinol Metab. 2014;99:3148–26.
90. Stanczyk FZ, Hapgood JP, Winer D, Mishell D Jr. Progestogens used in postmenopausal hormone therapy: differences in their pharmacological properties, intracellular actions, and clinical effects. Endocr Rev. 2013;34(2):171–208.
91. Gompel A. Micronized progesterone and its impact on the endometrium and breast vs. progestogens. Climacteric. 2012;15(1):18–25.
92. Mann E, Singer D, Pitkin J, Panay N, Hunter MS. Psychosocial adjustment in women with premature menopause: a cross-sectional survey. Climacteric. 2012;15:481–9.
93. Thurston RC, El Khoudary SR, Tepper PG, et al. Trajectories of vasomotor symptoms and carotid intima media thickness in the study of Women's health across the nation. Stroke. 2016;47:12–7.
94. L'Hermite M. HRT optimization using transdermal estradiol plus micronized progesterone, a safer HRT. Climacteric. 2013;6(1):44–53.
95. Fournier A, Berrino F, Clavel-Chapelon F. Unequal risks for breast cancer associated with different hormone replacement therapies: results from the E3N cohort study. Breast Cancer Res Treat. 2008;107:103–11.
96. Lyytinen H, Pukkala E, Ylikorkala O. Breast cancer risk in postmenopausal women using estradiol-progestogen therapy. Obstet Gynecol. 2009;113:65–73.

97. Schnatz P, Pinkerton J, Utian W, Appt S, de Villiers T, Henderson V, Hodis H, Kaunitz A, Maki P, Manson J, Richard-Davis G, Santoro N, Sarrel P, Shifren J, Simon J, Stuenkel C. NAMS translational science symposium report a conversation about hormone therapy: is there an appropriate dose, route, and duration of use. Menopause. 2017;24(11):1221–35.
98. Kaunitz A, Manson J. Management of Menopausal Symptoms. Obstet Gynecol. 2015;126(4):859–76.
99. Chen W, Rosner B, Hankinson SE, Colditz GA, Willett WC. Moderate alcohol consumption during adult life, drinking patterns, and breast cancer risk. JAMA. 2011;306:1184–890.
100. US Preventive Services Task Force, Grossman DC, Curry SJ, Owens DK, et al. Hormone therapy for the primary prevention of chronic conditions in postmenopausal women: USPSTF Recommendation Statement. JAMA. 2017;318:2224–33.
101. Langer R, Simon J, Pines A, Lobo R, Hodis H, Pickar J, Archer D, Sarrel P, Utian W. Menopausal hormone therapy for primary prevention: why the USPSTF is wrong. Menopause. 2017;24(10):1101–12.
102. Lobo R, Davis S, De Villiers T, et al. Prevention of diseases after menopause. Climacteric. 2014;17:540–56.
103. Walsh JM, Pignone M. Drug treatment of hyperlipidemia in women. JAMA. 2004;291:2243–52.
104. Petretta M, Costanzo P, Perrone-Filardi P. Impact of gender in primary prevention of coronary heart disease with statin therapy: a meta-analysis. Int J Cardiol. 2010;138:25–31.
105. Brughts JJ, Yetkin T, Hoeks SE. The benefits of statins in people without established cardiovascular disease but with cardiovascular risk factors: meta-analysis of randomized controlled trials. BMJ. 2009;338:b2376.
106. Berger JS, Roncaglioni C, Avanzini F. Aspirin for the primary prevention of cardiovascular events in women and men: a sex-specific meta-analysis of randomized controlled trials. JAMA. 2006;295:306–13.
107. Ridker PM, Cook NR, Lee IM. A randomized trial of low-dose aspirin in the primary prevention of cardiovascular disease in women. NEJM. 2005;352:1293–304.
108. Utian WH. Psychosocial and socioeconomic burden of vasomotor symptoms in menopause: a comprehensive review. Health Qual Life Outcomes. 2005;3(47):1–10.
109. Miller VM, Mitchell Harman S. An update on hormone therapy in postmenopausal women: mini-review for the basic scientist. Am J Physiol Heart Circ Physiol. 2017;313(5):H1013–21.
110. Hodis HN, Mack WJ. Cardiovascular risk after withdrawal of hormone therapy. Menopause. 2018;25(4):365–7.
111. Tepper P, Randolph J, Jones B, et al. Trajectory patterns of vasomotor symptoms over the menopausal transition in the study of women's health across the nation. Menopause. 2013;20:1356.
112. Labrie F. Intracrinology and menopause: the science describing the cell-specific intracellular formation of estrogens and androgens from DHEA and their strictly local action and inactivation in peripheral tissues. Menopause. 2018;26(2):220–4.
113. Modi M, Dhillo W. Neurokinin 3 receptor antagonism: a novel treatment for menopausal hot flushes. Neuroendocrinology. 2018;109(3):242–8. https://doi.org/10.1159/000495889.
114. Thurston RC, Johnson BD, Shufelt CL, Braunstein GD, Berga SL, Stanczyk FZ, Pepine CJ, Bittner V, Reis SE, Thompson DV, Kelsey SF, Sopko G, Merz CN. Menopausal symptoms and cardiovascular disease mortality in the Women's Ischemia Syndrome Evaluation (WISE). Menopause. 2017;24(2):126–32.
115. Thurston RC, Chang Y, Barinas-Mitchell E, et al. Menopausal hot flashes and carotid intima media thickness among midlife women. Stroke. 2016;47:2910–5.
116. Mendelsohn ME, Karas RH. The protective effects of estrogen on the cardiovascular system. NEJM. 1999;340(23):1801–11.
117. Hodis HN, Mack WJ, Henderson VW, et al. Vascular effects of early versus late postmenopausal treatment with estradiol. NEJM. 2016;374(13):1221–31.
118. Baber RJ, Panay N, Fenton A, the IMS Writing Group. 2016 IMS recommendations on women's midlife health and menopause hormone therapy. Climacteric. 2016;19(2):109–50.

Replacement Hormone Therapy for Gender Dysphoria and Congenital Sexual Anomalies

Angelica Mareş Miceli

What is it about sexuality that makes it such a burning matter since the dawn of mankind? So much so that even kings had to "give their consent"? Religion called it "a sin". Legislators got involved. Why was Egon Schiele convicted for "crimes against morality" and his drawing burnt by a judge? Why was Oscar Wilde deprived of his freedom for his sexual orientation? Much was lost of humankind heritage because of society's attitude toward sex and gender.

Today's human society came a long way. Medical knowledge progressed incredibly and so did social and cultural norms. In these days, on most places on the planet, there is acceptance. Still, gender issues take a center stage, often inflaming the social and political milieu everywhere. So how informed and prepared is the medical community to deal with these issues?

It used to be binary, male or female, mutually exclusive states. Yin or Yang. Now that approach is called "traditional" and "outdated." In today's society, is more and more accepted a perception of gender identity as a continuum, a spectrum going from male to female with other identities in between, a "gender fluidity" where one's sexual identity is not merely defined and dominated by one's genitals [1]. "Binary thinking" is opposed and replaced by a more inclusive, expanded view, creating a safer environment for the patients. There is a plethora of books and articles published in the last decade or so, approaching the subject from different angles, from guidelines to definitions to practical advices for clinicians.

A. Mareş Miceli (✉)
New York Medical College, Westchester Medical Center, Valhalla, NY, USA
e-mail: amares@nymc.edu

L. Deligdisch-Schor, A. Mareş Miceli (eds.), *Hormonal Pathology of the Uterus*, Advances in Experimental Medicine and Biology 1242,
https://doi.org/10.1007/978-3-030-38474-6_7

1 Definitions

At this point, maybe a *dictionary of terms* is necessary. What is gender dysphoria? Is it the same as transgender? Do all gender-diverse persons have gender dysphoria? Are all people with gender dysphoria transgender? Standardized terminology for healthcare providers was developed and is in use.

To begin with, *gender dysphoria* is a new diagnosis in the American Psychiatric Association's Diagnostic and Statistical Manual of Mental Disorders, Fifth Edition (DSM-5), replacing the DSM-IV diagnosis of gender identity disorder [2]. It is defined as a *marked incongruence between the patient's experienced or expressed gender and his or her assigned gender at birth.* In other words, gender dysphoria is a distress associated with one's own sense of self/gender identity and one's gender phenotype and assigned gender role due to that phenotype. For a clinician to diagnose gender dysphoria, the patient has to report at least 6 months of significant distress or impairment in social or occupational areas, due to at least two out of these six criteria:

1. Marked incongruence between one's experienced or expressed gender and primary and/or secondary sex characteristics
2. Strong desire to be rid of one's primary and/or secondary sex characteristics
3. Strong desire for the primary and/or secondary sex characteristics of the other gender
4. Strong desire to be of the other gender
5. Strong desire to be treated as the other gender
6. Strong conviction that one has the typical feelings and reactions of the other gender

According to a number of publications, there is a dramatic increase in gender dysphoria cases in the last decade or so, especially due to increased number of young people with gender dysphoria seeking medical attention for gender-confirming therapies [3–6].

The list of definitions and gender-related terminology is long and continuously evolving [7]; here are some of the most important ones.

A *transgender* is a person whose gender identity or expression differs from their sex assigned at birth.

Gender identity is an internalized sense of self as being male, female, or elsewhere along or outside the gender continuum. Some people have complex identities and may identify as agender, gender nonbinary, genderqueer, or gender fluid.

Sexual orientation is a term describing an enduring physical and emotional attraction to another group; sexual orientation is distinct from gender identity and is defined by the individual. Gender identity is distinct from sexual orientation, sex development, and external gender expression (display of gender identity through behavior, voice, interests, or appearance such as clothing or hairstyle).

A *transgender female* is a transgender person designated as male at birth.

A *transgender male* is a transgender person designated as female at birth.

It is beyond the purpose of this chapter to exhaust the entire list of terms, but this is one last definition for a historical term: transsexual. A *transsexual* is a transgender person seeking medical or surgical therapy in order to affirm their gender.

Transgender and gender-diverse persons may have gender dysphoria (i.e., distress related to this incongruence) or not.

2 Therapeutic Approach

Today there is an ever-growing body of research about gender dysphoric or gender incongruent individuals and the gender-affirming therapy. Therapeutic approaches for gender dysphoric patients include not only hormonal therapy and surgery but also facial hair removal, interventions for the modification of speech and communication, and other changes in gender expression and role, by living partially or totally in the desired gender role. Psychotherapy is another important constituent part of therapy for gender dysphoric patients; it includes not only the individual but also the couple, the family, or even group therapy. All of these procedures have been accepted as being medically sound and necessary by the WPATH (World Professional Association for Transgender Health) [8].

Medical care for gender dysphoria and for that matter for certain congenital sexual anomalies requiring it, is very complex and long in duration, with life-altering consequences. It starts with creating an optimal clinical environment and performing a complete medical evaluation, ideally multidisciplinary, including physical and mental exam. Past medical practices involved a succession of psychological assessment followed by hormonal treatment followed by surgery. For cases of gender dysphoria, the current standard of care is to allow every transgender person to seek only those treatments they wish, either medical or surgical or both, in order to affirm their own gender identity [9].

Aside from hormonal therapies, a wide range of *surgical interventions* are available to transgender patients, such as feminizing vaginoplasties, masculinizing phalloplasty or scrotoplasty, metaoidioplasty (clitoral release or enlargement), masculinizing chest surgery, facial feminization procedures, or voice surgery, to name only few.

3 Hormonal Therapy: Introduction

Primary medical intervention for gender affirmation is hormonal therapy. Feminizing and masculinizing hormone therapies are partially irreversible treatments, used to facilitate the development of secondary sex characteristics of the experienced gender.

Feminizing hormone therapy for the transgender female includes estrogen (17-beta estradiol) and progestogens, together with antiandrogens (spironolactone and 5-alpha reductase inhibitors); their role is to decrease the serum testosterone level to less than 50 ng/dL while maintaining a serum estradiol level of less than 200 pg/mL. This hormonal therapy may reduce muscle mass, decrease libido and terminal hair growth, and increase breast development and fat redistribution. In clinical studies, voice change was not an expected effect. Additional risks for feminizing hormonal therapy include breast cancer, prolactinoma, cardiovascular or cerebrovascular disease, cholelithiasis, and hypertriglyceridemia; however, these risks are rare or incompletely studied [10].

Masculinizing hormone therapy for the transgender male includes testosterone to increase serum levels to 320–1000 ng/dL. Anticipated changes include acne, weight gain, scalp hair loss, facial and body hair growth, voice deepening, vaginal atrophy, clitoromegaly, and increased muscle mass. Patients receiving masculinizing hormone therapy are at risk of erythrocytosis, as well as other possible metabolic effects, but to date there is limited data about outcomes as death, thromboembolic disease, stroke, osteoporosis, liver toxicity, or myocardial infarction [11–14].

There are many facets to consider when contemplating hormonal treatment. Active hormone-sensitive malignancy is an absolute contraindication to gender-affirming hormone treatment. Patients who are older, use tobacco, or have severe chronic disease, current or previous venous thrombo-embolism, or a history of hormone-sensitive malignancy should benefit from subspecialty consultation followed by individualized dosing regimens. In general, the benefits and risks of treatment should be carefully explained and weighed against the risks of no action (such as suicidal ideation) [15].

Not all gender dysphoric persons need or seek hormonal treatment; however, those who receive it, generally report an improved quality of life, with reduced anxiety levels and higher self-esteem [15, 16]. Gender-affirming hormone therapy mostly includes commonly used substances, familiar to most prescribers due to their use in the management of menopause, contraception, hirsutism, male pattern baldness, or abnormal uterine bleeding. Not only subspecialty clinicians, such as obstetricians-gynecologists and endocrinologists, but also primary care physicians may evaluate gender dysphoria and prescribe applicable hormone therapy or monitor well-being and provide referrals.

Hormone therapy with estrogens and antiandrogens or testosterone is generally safe but can be irreversible. Surgical therapy for gender affirmation has its own risks, not to mention its irreversible character, and should be done only if patients have sufficient mental ability to give informed consent. That is why guidelines are necessary and a team of healthcare providers should be consulted on issues like when to start the treatment, what treatment should be offered, and how often should the patients receive it.

Updated guidelines of the Endocrine Society on transgender medical care, cosponsored by the American Association of Clinical Endocrinologists, American Society of Andrology, European Society for Paediatric Endocrinology, European Society of Endocrinology, Pediatric Endocrine Society, and the World Professional Association for Transgender Health, include the following key points:

1. Prepubertal patients displaying gender dysphoria should not receive hormone therapy.
2. Clinicians should inform their patients about different options for preservation of fertility, before starting puberty-suppression treatments (in adolescents) or hormonal therapy.
3. In adolescents, treatment with GnRH analogues for hormone suppression should start after physical changes of puberty are present.
4. Clinicians should evaluate and treat other medical conditions patients may have that can be exacerbated by an eventual hormone therapy.
5. In cases of patients who need high doses of steroids to suppress their own body synthesis of sex hormones, surgical removal of gonads may be considered.
6. Hormone therapy should be followed by long-term care, with all patients having regular monitoring of prolactin levels, bone loss, cardiovascular and metabolic disorders and evidently, cancer screening [17].

4 Hormonal Therapy for the Transgender Female

Hormonal therapy for the transgender female, so-called "feminizing hormone therapy" or the male-to-female type (MTF) has the purpose to change the secondary sexual characteristics from androgynous into feminine (i.e., development of breasts, feminine pattern of hair, fat and muscle distribution, etc.) while suppressing the male secondary sex characteristics.

The medications used for MTF therapy include estrogens, antiandrogens, progestogens, and GnRH (gonadotropin-releasing hormone) modulators. If estrogens are administered postpuberty, it cannot undo many of the changes produced by naturally occurring puberty; these may necessitate sex reassignment surgery and other treatments in order to be reversed.

There are several contraindications for feminizing hormone therapy, absolute and relative. The absolute contraindications are an estrogen-sensitive malignancy or a medical history of it (i.e., breast, pituitary) and history of or increased risk of thromboembolism, unless currently treated. Relative contraindications include a family history of breast cancer and thromboembolic disease, liver and kidney pathology, heart disease or risk factors for heart disease, strokes, hypercoagulability states.

The mainstay of MTF hormonal therapy is estrogen, administered as 17-beta estradiol (chemical product identical to the naturally synthesized estrogen by the ovary) in a manner similar to the treatment of agonadal states (congenital, such as Turner syndrome, or surgically acquired) or postmenopausal states. Conjugated estrogens and ethinylestradiol are rarely used, due to their high risk for cardiovascular pathology. The main effect of estrogen therapy is "chemical castration", that is suppressing the testosterone level by ~95%; this effect is achieved usually by levels of 200 pg/mL of estradiol. Obviously, dosages of estrogens can be reduced after an orchiectomy or sex reassignment surgery, when testosterone suppression is no longer needed [17].

When testosterone levels are inadequately suppressed by estradiol alone, antiandrogens such as spironolactone and 5-alpha reductase inhibitors (finasteride and dutasteride) can be used to further reduce or even suppress the effects of testosterone with the consequent change in the male secondary sexual characteristics. Antiandrogens can also be used alone in patients who want to first explore reduced testosterone levels before starting estrogen therapy or in cases of absolute contraindications to estrogen therapy. In these cases, some patients may experience hot flashes and low energy. As in the case of long-term androgen blockade without estrogen replacement in men treated for prostate cancer resulting in bone loss, the same effects would be expected in the similar treatment of transgender individuals [15].

Progestogens don't yet have a defined role in feminizing hormone therapies; their use is controversial at best. To date, there have been no studies and no evidence pointing to the effects, positive or negative, of progestogens. There are two types of progestogens: progesterone, the natural hormone, and progestins, which are synthetic progestogens. At high doses, progestogens have antiandrogenic effect (due to their antigonadotropic effect with subsequent suppression of testosterone levels). Clinical research about the use of progestogens in transgender women is limited, but there are many claims about their benefic effects (i.e., improved breast development, mood, and libido). Aside from these positive effects, progestogens can have adverse effects, ranging from sedation and mood changed, to increased risk of cardiovascular disease (when added to estrogen therapy) and frequency of some benign tumors (i.e., prolactinomas, meningiomas, etc.). In general, the response of transgender women to progestogens therapy is very variable, with some responding favorably, while others had negative effects [15]. Some researchers recommend that, due to their potential adverse effects and the lack of scientific evidence in favor of their beneficial effect, progestogen therapy in transgender women should not be used or at most be used only for a limited period of time (2–3 years) [18]. Equally, other researchers maintained that the risks of progestogens in transgender women are likely minimal, and due to their theoretical benefits, should be used.

GnRH modulators are substances capable of completely shutting down gonadal sex hormone production; they can decrease testosterone levels by about 95% which is equivalent to the surgical castration state. They tend to have very few side effects when administered together with estrogen-replacement therapy.

There are many physical changes as a result of hormone-replacement therapy in transgender women: breast development (with potential for lactation), skin changes (thinning of the skin, with accumulation of subcutaneous fat and reduced sebaceous gland activity), eye and hair changes, reduction in the muscle mass with redistribution, bone and joints changes. However, characteristics already established after puberty will not be affected (height, facial hair, voice features, etc.). Aside from physical effects, there are also mood changes, libido changes, and neurological changes.

In terms of adverse effects, hormonal therapy increases the risk of thromboembolic events (deep vein thrombosis, pulmonary thromboembolism), the risk of liver toxicity, may cause development of prolactinomas, and results in changes of cancer risks, protecting against breast cancer [19] and prostate cancer [20, 21].

5 Hormonal Therapy for the Transgender Male

Hormonal therapy for the transgender male, so-called "masculinizing hormone therapy" or the female-to-male type (FTM), has the purpose of adjusting the secondary sex characteristics to those of the desired sex/experienced gender, in this case, the development of male secondary sex characteristics (voice deepening and a masculine pattern of hair, fat, and muscle distribution) while suppressing or minimizing the female secondary sex characteristics.

The medications used for FTM therapy include androgens (namely testosterone) and for prepubertal patients, puberty-suppression therapy with a GnRH analogue (Lupron, Supprelin). As is the case with estrogens, if testosterone is administered postpuberty, it cannot undo many of the changes produced by naturally occurring puberty; these may necessitate surgery and other treatments to be reversed.

There are several contraindications for masculinizing hormone therapy, absolute (pregnancy) and relative (polycythemia, liver disease, coronary artery disease, cardiac failure, bleeding disorders, history of breast cancer, androgen-sensitive epilepsy, migraines, sleep apnea, renal failure, or severe hypertension susceptible to sodium retention and fluid overload, history of violent behavior, and acne, mild to severe).

Many available formulations exist for testosterone, from the natural hormone to dihydrotestosterone and synthetic androgens (e.g., nandrolone), as well as many ways of administration; it can be injected, administered transdermal, oral, sublingual or as skin implants. In practice, most commonly used is parenteral testosterone, injected intramuscularly or subcutaneously, or transdermal testosterone 1% (incompletely studied and less used) [22, 23]. In general, changes begin after 1–6 months of therapy and stabilize after about 1–3 years of treatments.

Menstruation-suppression therapies can be used concomitantly with testosterone therapy or prior to its initiation and include combined oral contraceptives (ethinyl estradiol with variable doses of progestin), depot medroxyprogesterone, or levonorgestrel-releasing intrauterine IUD (Mirena).

Antiestrogens like aromatase inhibitors (e.g., anastrozole) or selective estrogen receptor modulators (e.g., tamoxifen) can be used to diminish the effects of high levels of endogenous estrogen in transgender men. In addition, due to the fact that growth process is mediated by estrogen, in adolescents who didn't conclude their growth (bone epiphysis are not closed yet), antiestrogens can help prevent reaching an increased final height as well as hip widening. Finasteride and dutasteride (5α-Reductase inhibitors) can also be used in the FTM hormonal treatment, to slow or prevent scalp hair loss and excessive body hair growth in transgender men taking testosterone.

The end result of FTM hormonal therapy consists of multiple physical and psychological changes, from skin and hair changes to reproductive changes, from cardiovascular to metabolic, neurological and mood changes. Some of these changes are reversible (redistribution of body fat, from a gynoid to an android pattern, increased musculature, increased red blood cell count, increased libido, cessation of ovulation and menstruation, etc.) while others are not (deepening of the voice, growth of facial and body hair, growth spurt and closure of growth plates if hormones were given before the end of puberty, clitoromegaly frequently at apex within 2–3 years of therapy, breast atrophy—mainly due to the loss of adipose tissue of the breast.).

5.1 Effects of Hormonal Therapy for the Transgender Male: Histological Aspects

Hormonal treatment with testosterone induces a hypoestrogenic state and, in a dose-dependent fashion, has an effect on vaginal tissue consisting of atrophy and increased vaginal pH, consequently increasing the risk of infections (vaginitis, cystitis, and cervicitis). Furthermore, the thinned, atrophic vaginal mucosa is more susceptible to trauma which may result in dyspareunia (painful vaginal intercourse).

Menses should cease within 5–6 months of testosterone therapy (often sooner). Cessation of menses is driven by a combination of testosterone effect on ovaries, consisting of induced ovulation suppression (which may be incomplete), and endometrial atrophy. Initially thought that exogenous testosterone produces a milieu of "unopposed" estrogen by the way of aromatization to estrogen and also, possibly, by inducing an anovulatory state, thus theoretically increasing the risk of endometrial hyperplasia and carcinoma, some long-term data do not support this risk [24]. Literature shows only one such case report [25] and in fact, few more studies show that the risk of endometrial hyperplasia and cancer is low due mainly to the fact that transgender men develop endometrial atrophy while on androgen treatment [26, 27].

However, if prior to initiation of testosterone therapy, the patient had a history of abnormal cycles (e.g., menorrhagia, metrorrhagia) cessation of menses may take longer than 6 months, and if menstrual bleeding continues for more than 6–12 months, the condition is described as "abnormal uterine bleeding" (AUB). AUB may be explained by prior existence of underlying uterine pathology. Most common causes include endometrial polyps, adenomyosis, leiomyomas, endometrial hyperplasia, and malignancy. These conditions should be investigated by imaging (sonogram, transabdominal ultrasound, CT scan or MRI, etc.) and endometrial biopsy. Other causes for AUB can be pregnancy (of course, ruling out of a pregnancy should be mandatory before initiation of testosterone therapy), ovarian causes (malignancy, ovarian dysfunction, etc.), or iatrogenic causes.

After long-term androgen therapy not only lower gynecological tract organs but also ovaries develop some pathological conditions. While some case reports of ovarian cancer in transgender men were published [28, 29], there is no evidence to suggest an increased risk of ovarian cancer in transgender men on androgen therapy. In terms of histological changes in the ovaries after testosterone treatment, there are not many studies done to date.

The classical concept is that administration of androgens causes ovarian histological features suggestive of polycystic ovarian disease (PCOD). In a study conducted by Dr. Deligdisch [30, 31], the effects of exogenously administered testosterone on ovaries was studied on a group of 19 transgender men who underwent bilateral salpingo-oophorectomy and compared to those in an age-matched group of 12 patients who underwent pelvic surgery for nonendocrine reasons. The most significant findings in the transgender men's ovaries in this study included enlarged or borderline enlarged ovaries, multiple ovarian cystic follicles in various stages of growth and atresia (89.5% of the patients), diffuse ovarian stroma hyperplasia (84.2% of the patients), collagenization of the outer ovarian cortex (68.42% of the patients), and luteinization of stromal cells (26.3% of the patients). Clinical and microscopic findings of the 19 androgen-treated transgender men are shown in Table 1. These data suggested that exogenous testosterone leads to development of morphologic features similar to PCOS (Figs. 1 and 2).

These findings are supported by newer studies [26]. Dr. Grynberg et al. conducted an analysis of 112 transgender men who received exogenous androgens for at least 6 months prior to undergoing hystero-salpingo-oophorectomy. Moreover, they analyzed specimens from additional 100 mastectomies which allowed them a study of the breast tissue from the same cohort. Their main findings include an increased mean ovarian volume, with histological characteristics of PCOS defined as >12 antral follicles per ovary (79.5% of the patients), endometrial atrophy (45% of the patients), marked reduction of breast glandular tissue, and increase of fibrous connective tissue without atypical hyperplasia or carcinoma (93% of the patients).

These data confirm the associations between long-term androgen administration and abnormalities in ovarian architecture with macroscopic and microscopic characteristics of PCOS, together with an increased risk of endometrial atrophy and also development of fibrotic breast tissue with marked glandular reduction.

6 Cancer Screening After Hormonal Treatment in Transgender Persons

As a general commonsense rule, an ongoing and thorough medical and surgical history is essential to determine an individual patient's screening needs, and this is the rule that should apply to transgender persons undergoing hormonal treatment.

There are not many long-term follow-up studies for this cohort of patients, but existing studies showed that there are not major differences in this category,

Table 1 Clinical and microscopic findings of 19 androgen-treated transgender men

Patient No.	Age (years)	Hirsute	Collagenization of outer cortex	Cystic follicles		Luteinized theca interna	Corpus luteum	Corpora albicantia	Luteinized stromal cells	Stromal hyperplasia	Endometrium		Polycystic ovaries
				Multiple	>6 mm in diameter						Proliferative	Inactive	
1	29		+	+	–	+	–	–	+	+		+	Yes
2	23	2+	+	+	–	+	–	–	+	++		+	Yes
3	20	2+	–	+	+	–	+	+	+	–		+	No
4	30	2+	+	+	–	+	–	–	–	++	+ hyp		Yes
5	38		+	+	–	–	–	+	–	+	+		Yes
6	30		–	+	+	–	–	+	–	–	+		No
7	31		+	+	+	+	–	–	+	+	+ hyp		Yes
8	26		–	+	–	–	–	–	–	–	+		No
9	24		+	+	–	–	–	+	–	+	+		Yes
10	23		–	–	–	–	–	–	–	+	+		No
11	32	1+	–	+	+	+	–	–	–	+	+		Yes
12	20		+	+	–	–	–	–	+	+		+	Yes
13	24	2+	+	+	–	–	–	–	–	+		+	Yes
14	25	3+	+	–	–	–	–	+	–	+++		+	No
15	24		–	+	–	–	+	–	–	+		+	No
16	25		+	+	–	–	–	–	–	+	+		Yes
17	45		+	+	–	–	+	–	–	+	+		Yes
18	20	1 +	+	+	–	+	–	–	–	+	+		Yes
19	20	1 +	+	+	+	+	–	–	–	+	+ hyp		Yes
n			13	17	5	7	3	5	5	16	12	7	13 and 1 with stromal hyperplasia

+, present; –, absent; hyp, hyperplastic

compared to controls. However, there are many limitations to this studies and insufficient evidence exists as to assess an increase or decrease of the overall organ-specific cancer risk [32].

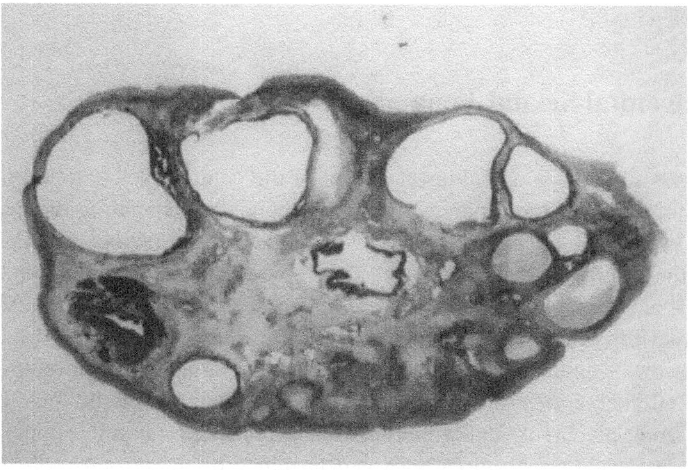

Fig. 1 Section of polycystic ovary in androgen-treated patient showing multiple cystic follicles distributed beneath a thickened collagenized external ovarian cortex. Whole mount, ×2.5

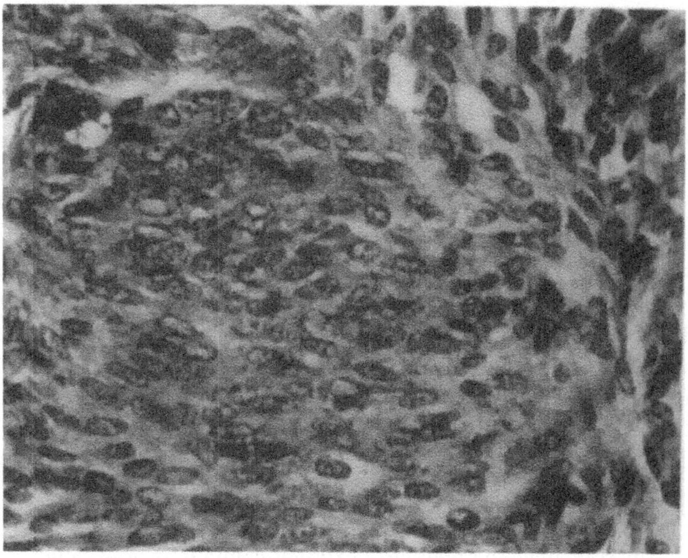

Fig. 2 Cystic follicle of androgen-treated patient lined by granulosa and prominent luteinized theca cells. Hematoxylin and eosin stain. Magnification, ×120

This being the reality, primary care providers should conduct an organ-based routine cancer screening for all transgender patients in accordance with current guidelines, keeping in mind that if the patient still has an organ that meets the criteria for screening (e.g. did not undergo mastectomy, oophorectomy, or hysterectomy, etc.) based on risk factors, symptoms, or general screening recommendations, this patient should undergo screening regardless of exogenous hormonal treatment.

7 Congenital Sexual Anomalies

The process of embryological development of the genital tract starts in the fourth week of intrauterine development and is very complex, depending on an intricate series of events influenced, directly or indirectly, by many factors, such as expression of transcription factors, germ cell development and migration from the yolk sac, X chromosome integrity, and secretion of sex steroid hormones. Male and female tract reproductive development starts from an undifferentiated mesoderm known as the "genital ridge"; afterwards, the urogenital ridges develop into the kidneys, adrenal cortex areas, gonads, and reproductive tracts. Initially, both Wolffian (male precursor) and Müllerian (female precursor) ducts develop. Initiation of embryo's development into a male is determined by the presence of SRY gene ("sex-determining region on the Y chromosome" gene) either in a male genotype or in some cases, in an XX genotype in which the SRY region was retained as a result of a translocation.

There are many congenital sexual anomalies and even more attempts to classify them, which at best are controversial [33–37]. Although it is beyond the scope of this chapter to extenuate the classification of congenital sexual anomalies, a brief discussion is necessary.

Among the most commonly clinically encountered sexual congenital anomalies, there are: *agenesis or hypoplasia of a urogenital ridge* (most common form in this class is the Mayer–Rokitansky–Küster–Hauser syndrome), ovarian hypoplasia (aka Turner syndrome), agenesis and dysgenesis of the ovary (histopathologically indistinguishable from Turner syndrome), androgen insensitivity syndrome (aka testicular feminization syndrome), hermaphroditism, and pseudohermaphroditism; also, congenital abnormalities of the human female genital tract occurring when the paired Müllerian ducts fail to fuse or the subsequent septum fails to resorb, yield an entire spectrum of uterine anomalies: unicornuate uterus, uterus didelphys, bicornuate uterus, septate uterus, arcuate uterus, absent vagina, septate vagina, ambiguous genitalia, etc.

Advances in understanding of sex determination, sex differentiation, and psychosexual development led to adoption of new terms and newer classifications. The complex group of congenital disorders resulting in the phenotypic appearance of atypical (formerly called "ambiguous") external genitalia is now called "disorders of sexual development" (DSD) [38–41]. In brief, DSD include XX, DSD (e.g., virilizing congenital adrenal hyperplasia, maternal androgen secreting tumor, ovotesticular disorders), XY DSD (e.g., impaired testosterone synthesis, Denys–Drash syndrome, etc.), sex chromosome DSD (Turner syndrome, Klinefelter syndrome, mosaicism, triple XXX syndrome), XX/XY disorder of gonadal development (complete gonadal dysgenesis, partial gonadal dysgenesis, gonadal regression, ovotesticular DSD), XY persistent Müllerian duct syndrome, and malformation syndromes.

The birth of an infant with atypical genitalia and underlying disorder of sexual development (DSD) is cause of enormous anxiety for parents and presents unique challenges with respect to sex assignment, parental education, and medical management. Although many of these patients are diagnosed in infancy due to the phenotypical presentation that warrants immediate evaluation, some patients with DSD are diagnosed later in life, when they seek medical attention for puberty disorders. In all cases, there are many aspects to be addressed, including parental issues, ethical and social considerations, medical and surgical treatments; therefore, a multidisciplinary approach including neonatologists, pediatric endocrinologists, urologists, surgeons, gynecologists, radiologists, geneticists, etc. is always recommended.

The historic approach for the management of these patients consists of early surgery for "correcting the external genitalia" together with eventual gonadectomy, all done in the name of "matching the assigned gender." Recently though, the process of "gender assignment" considers many factors, including a well-established (whenever possible) etiological diagnosis of the DSD, options for fertility preservation, eventual need for replacement hormonal therapy during puberty and finally, delayed, elective surgical treatments.

7.1 Hormonal Treatment: General Considerations

In terms of hormonal treatment for different congenital sexual anomalies, there are few generally accepted standard approaches. With the exception of congenital adrenal hyperplasia, hormonal treatment is directed toward pubertal induction (in cases of hypogonadism), started around 10–13 years of age, and hormone replacement therapy started at different ages, with the declared purpose of gender identity reinforcement, secondary sexual characteristics development, and psychosexual health promotion.

Patients with adrenal insufficiency at presentation need immediate replacement therapy with hydrocortisone. For the purpose of puberty induction, hormonal therapy with sex steroids is controversial in terms of time for initiation, doses, and regimen, but most clinicians agree that hormonal treatment should be started around 11–12 years of age, with low doses which can be progressively increased.

For patients with female gender identity and a uterus, pubertal induction is attempted with low doses of estrogen, gradually increasing the dose in a way that mimics natural puberty process. After few years of estrogen therapy or after initiation of menses (or breakthrough bleeding), progesterone is added to the therapeutic regimen, in order to mimic the physiological hormonal cycle. Of note is the situation where the patient lacks a uterus; in these cases, there is no need to add progesterone to the existing hormonal treatment. Similarly, for patients with male gender identity, hormonal treatments with testosterone in different doses and ways of administration are available for puberty induction.

In cases of patients over 50 years of age with gonadal failure, there is no consensus about optimal hormonal replacement therapies. It was suggested that agonadal women should be treated in a similar way as symptomatic perimenopausal women, with estrogen replacement, with a recommendation for screening mammography. For male patients with gonadal failure, indefinite testosterone therapy is currently advised with the recommendation for prostate exams and PSA testing according to the existing guidelines.

Following are some of the most common congenital anomalies and details of their specific treatments.

7.2 *Patients with 45, X0/46, XY and 46, XX/46, XY Mosaicism*

In cases of 45,X0/46,XY mosaicism (mixed gonadal dysgenesis), patients present with dysgenetic testes or streak gonads, hypoplastic and unilateral. External genitalia are variable, asymmetrical (possible unilateral cryptorchidism), rarely fully male or fully female. Management of these patients includes gonadal biopsy for diagnostic confirmation. Usually, these dysgenetic gonads carry a high risk of gonadoblastoma, requiring gonadectomy.

Patients with 46,XX/46,XY mosaicism may present with both a testicle and an ovary (in the same individual) or a mixture of ovarian and testicular tissue in the same gonad (ovotestis) (Fig. 3); in older classification, these patients were known as

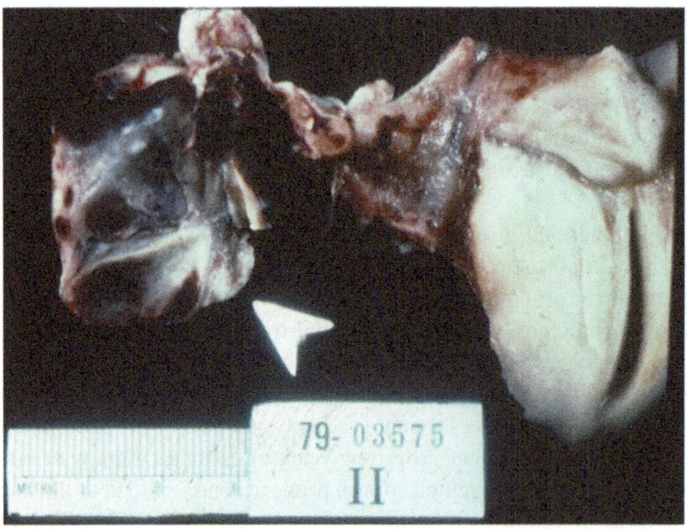

Fig. 3 Ovotestis in true hermaphrodite

"true hermaphrodites." It should be mentioned that ovotesticular cases also include pure gonadal dysgenesis: 46,XX ovotesticular DSD (33% of all ovotesticular cases) and 46,XY ovotesticular DSD (7% of ovotesticular cases or chimerism). The diagnosis of hermaphroditism is based entirely on the gonads; the external genitalia phenotype is variable and ranges from entirely female to entirely male, with intermediate phenotypes characterized by ambiguous genitalia. Management of these patients includes gonadal biopsy for diagnostic confirmation. If ovotestis is present, resection of testicular tissue has to be considered, due to an existing 3% risk of malignant transformation.

Compared to the general population, patients with DSD have an increased risk of developing germ cell tumors. There is a number of risk factors generally believed to be responsible for these tumors increased incidence, and they include (a) the presence of GBY (Gonadoblastoma on the Y chromosome) region and the gene TSPY, most recent genetic candidate; (b) expression of the embryonic germ cell markers (OCT3/4 and KITL) in patients older than 1-year of age; (c) the anatomical location of the gonads. Most common tumor types encountered in dysgenetic gonads are CIS/IGCNU (carcinoma in situ/intratubular germ cell neoplasia unclassified) in a dysgenetic testis and gonadoblastoma.

Gonadoblastomas, first described by Robert Scully in 1953, are rare neoplasms composed of germ cell and sex cord–stromal derivatives; they are almost always seen in patients with dysgenetic gonads or undescended testis. Approximately 40% are bilateral, small (sometimes apparent only microscopically), yellow brown, sometimes with calcifications. Microscopically, gonadoblastomas show a mixture of primitive germ cells resembling seminoma and sex-cord cells resembling Sertoli and granulosa cells. Leydig cells or luteinized stromal cells are frequently noted, as well as calcifications (present in ~80% of cases). As a matter of fact, coarse calcifications in an invasive germ cell tumor should raise the suspicion of origin from gonadoblastoma. About 50% of these patients eventually develop invasive seminoma, and ~10% more develop other germ cell tumors. The prognosis for patients with pure gonadoblastoma is excellent, but in those cases with a malignant germ cell component, the prognosis will depend on the features of the invasive tumor.

7.3 Turner Syndrome and Variants: (45,X-) and 45, X0/46,XX Mosaicism

Patients with Turner syndrome and variants (45,X; monosomy X) and 45,X0/46,XX mosaicism present with gonadal dysgenesis in ~90% of the cases. Internal genitalia consist of variable degree of development of the Müllerian structures, while the phenotype is classically female, with pterigium coli, short stature.

Clinically, patients with Turner syndrome present with ovarian failure and amenorrhea. Histologically, the typical ovary in monosomy X is a streak gonad (Fig. 4). Grossly, the ovary is a small, flat ovoid structure; microscopically, it consists prin-

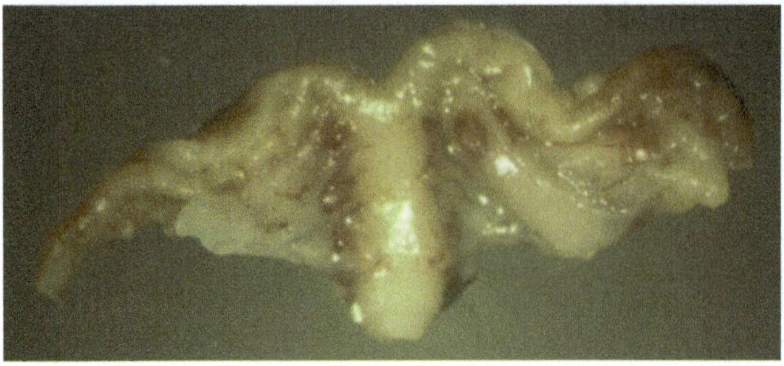

Fig. 4 Streak gonads in a patient with Turner syndrome

cipally of scant ovarian cortical stroma that may contain scattered primitive sex cord structures. Oocytes are not present due to an accelerated loss, of unknown cause, after the 18th week of fetal life or over the immediate postnatal period.

Patients with Turner syndrome may remain undiagnosed until puberty, when physical growth and sexual maturation are noted to lag behind the norm. Only approximately 5–10% of patients with Turner syndrome will have spontaneous pubertal development and menstrual periods; therefore, it is very important to make an early diagnosis of Turner syndrome. This will allow the timely initiation of appropriate hormonal therapy necessary to achieve normal growth and to induce puberty.

Hormonal treatment for these patients include recombinant growth hormone (if the patient has short stature) and steroid therapy for induction of puberty and replacement (most patients have variable degrees of hypergonadotropic hypogonadism).

The hormone replacement therapy includes estrogen and progesterone. Use of estrogen alone is associated with an increased risk of endometrial hyperplasia and neoplasia. On the endometrium, estrogen effects are time-dependent, resulting initially in an "irregular proliferative endometrium" (for a detailed description of this pathology, see Chap. 8). If a prolonged estrogen-only therapy is used in prepubertal patients with Turner syndrome with an infantile uterus, endometrial carcinoma may develop, frequently of endometrioid type, hormone receptor positive and with a favorable prognosis. Figure 5 shows a case of a 19-year-old patient with Turner syndrome who received long-term unopposed estrogen therapy and subsequently developed endometrioid endometrial adenocarcinoma.

To decrease the risk of endometrial neoplasia development due to therapy with estrogen alone, progesterone is usually added to the regimen. Although this is the rule, there are exceptions where endometrial biopsies from these patients show atypical endometrial hyperplasia and even endometrial carcinoma (for a detailed description of these pathological changes, see Chap. 8).

Endometrial neoplasia is not the only risk worth mentioning for Turner patients receiving hormonal therapy. These patients are also at an increased risk of developing gonadal neoplasia (e.g., gonadoblastoma and dysgerminoma) but these occurrences are independent of therapy and dependent on chromosomal constitution of

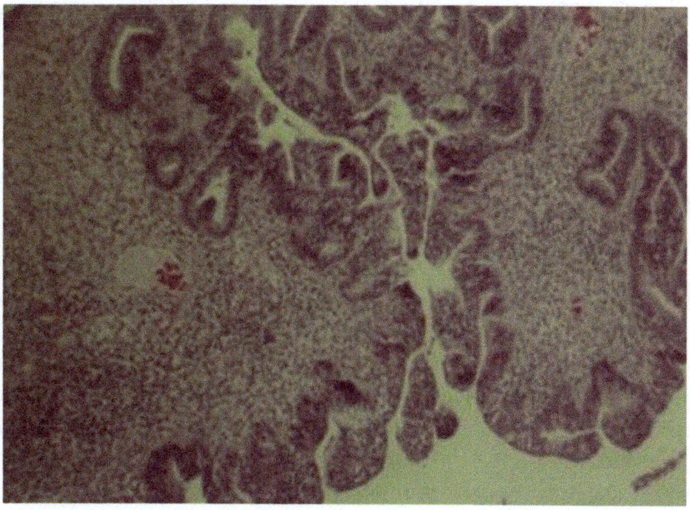

Fig. 5 Effect of 7-year duration estrogen replacement therapy on endometrial biopsy of a 19-year-old patient with Turner syndrome: well-differentiated adenocarcinoma, endometrioid type. H&E ×100

the patient: risk is increased only if their chromosomal constitution includes a Y chromosome with the SRY gene.

7.4 Klinefelter Syndrome

Patients with Klinefelter syndrome and variants (47,XXY etc.) have reduced body and pubic hair, gynecomastia in 40–75% of the cases, male external genitalia, small and firm (hyalinized) testes, and other features secondary to progressive androgen deficiency. Microscopically, sections from testis of a Klinefelter patient may show small and hyalinized seminiferous tubules, with focal atrophy and reduced number of intratubular germ cells; some tubules may show Sertoli cells only. Also noted are Leydig cell nodules, which due to surrounding tubular atrophy may appear hyperplastic.

These patients may require testosterone replacement therapy and eventual breast reduction surgery.

7.5 Androgen Insensitivity Syndrome

The androgen insensitivity syndrome patients have female phychosexual development; gender dysphoria is very rare. The typical patient with androgen insensitivity syndrome (partial or complete form) is a young girl presenting clinically with primary amenorrhea. These patients' gonads are functioning testes, which produce normal male hormones (androgens), but the lack of testosterone receptors results in a female phenotypic appearance. Androgen insensitivity syndrome is an X-linked recessive condition, confirmed by androgen receptor genetic sequencing.

These patients present with varied internal genitalia, from possible hypoplastic Wolffian structures in the partial forms of the syndrome to absent Wolffian structures and possible atrophic uterus in complete forms of the syndrome. Thus, internal genital organs may show a short vagina, ending in a blind pouch and absent cervix due to a blunted or suppressed uterine development. External genitalia are variable in partial syndrome while complete forms of the syndrome present as phenotypical females, with scant pubic and axillary hair.

Although most patients with complete androgen insensitivity syndrome have undescended, intra-abdominal testes, these are not dysgenetic; therefore, the risk of gonadoblastoma is lower, ~2% [42]. However, despite lower risks for development of neoplasia, these are not inexistent, making orchiectomy the standard of care. Although the ideal time for performing the surgery is still debatable, many advise in favor of delaying the procedure until after puberty, thus allowing for a spontaneous progression through puberty due to the metabolic pathway of peripheral testosterone aromatization into estrogen. At microscopic examination of removed testes, they may show Sertoli cell only tubules, nodular Sertoli cell masses, Leydig cell hyperplasia, and/or germ cell atypia or neoplasia [43].

For patients with complete androgen insensitivity syndrome, ongoing hormone replacement therapy with estrogen (or estrogen and progesterone, if the patient has a rudimentary uterus) is recommended, starting with a low dose which subsequently is progressively increased. There is some evidence, however debatable, that supports the idea that adding progesterone to the estrogen regimen has beneficial effects even in patients lacking a uterus, most important being reduction of long-term risk of breast cancer.

In rare cases of male patients with partial androgen sensitivity syndrome and undervirilization resulting in micropenis development, the treatment consists of testosterone and dihydrotestosterone, which can be used also topical, for the purpose of increasing penile length [44]. To date, there is no medical consensus about the efficacy of this therapy, dosages, and long-term outcomes.

7.6 Müllerian Agenesis

Developmental anomalies of the uterus can be due to one of the three mechanisms: failure of the Müllerian duct genesis (resulting in agenesis, bilateral hypoplasia, or unicornuate uterus), failure of Müllerian duct fusion (resulting in uterus didelphys and bicornuate uterus), or failure of the fused Müllerian wall to be resorbed (resulting in septate uterus).

Müllerian agenesis (also known as Müllerian aplasia or Mayer–Rokitansky–Küster–Hauser syndrome, or MRKH syndrome) is a severe anomaly with an incidence of 1 per 4500–5000 females. A combination of genetic and environmental factors is believed to contribute to the development of MRKH syndrome, although specific factors still remain unknown.

Müllerian duct is hypoplastic or absent, with different clinical expressions of varying severity. Isolated uterine and vaginal aplasia and hypoplasia is considered to be the "typical form of MRKH" syndrome. In the other instances, the "non-typical" form, there are coexisting urinary tract anomalies, ovarian dysgenesis, skeletal and cardiac malformations.

Patients with MRKH syndrome have no vagina but a shallow dimple lined by normal vaginal mucosa. A single midline uterine remnant may be present or uterine horns, with or without an endometrial cavity, may exist.

The MRKH syndrome patients also have well-developed ovaries, with normal function regarding ovulation and hormone secretion, although they may be found in atypical locations. Consequently, these patients, psychologically and physically 46,XX females, will have normal growth and development, but because uterine vestiges are nonfunctional, they will not menstruate. As is the case, the first clinical sign of MRKH syndrome is primary amenorrhea.

The initial evaluation of an adolescent patient with primary amenorrhea and normal height, breast development, body hair, and external genitalia includes a physical examination to assess for signs of appropriate or delayed puberty and laboratory tests (testosterone level, FSH level, and karyotype).

Imaging studies (transabdominal, translabial, or transrectal ultrasonography, MRI) typically will not identify a midline uterus; the primitive uterus may be located in the retroperitoneal space, with no mesentery, or may be located intraperitoneally, with a short mesentery. The fallopian tubes may or may not be present. The normal ovaries are always identified, together with the round ligament of the ovary attached to the adjacent uterine vestige [45]. If some active endometrium is present, the patient may experience cyclic or chronic abdominal pain. In these cases, laparoscopy may be useful for evaluation and management.

The differential diagnosis in these cases of patients presenting with primary amenorrhea and an absent vagina includes obstructing anomalies, such as imperforate hymen, transverse vaginal septum, or cervical atresia. Other conditions that need to be ruled out are androgen insensitivity syndrome and *CYP17A1* deficiency.

After establishing a correct diagnosis and conducting further investigation for any associated congenital anomalies, another important aspect of effective management of MRKH syndrome patients that has to be remembered is psychosocial counseling. The psychologic effect of depression and anxiety that such a diagnosis has on the patients (as well as on her family) should not be underestimated; patients should be referred to support groups and encouraged to connect with young women with the same diagnosis.

General surgical management of anatomic anomalies consists of an initial trial of vaginal dilatation and elongation, followed by the surgical creation (through many different techniques) of a neovagina. In cases in which surgical intervention is required, referrals to centers with this specific expertise should be considered for a successful result.

Fertility issues should also be discussed with patients with MRKH syndrome. These patients should be informed of the many alternatives available, from adoption to gestational carrier (surrogacy) and to newest technique, uterine transplantation.

Uterine transplants although still highly experimental, became a real treatment option for infertility of different causes. At the beginning of this decade, for patients with MRKH syndrome, the only available options to have a child were adoption or surrogacy. This situation was changed by the first childbirths following uterine transplantation from living donors in Gothenburg, Sweden, in September, 2013. It is this author's great honor to have personally witnessed and to remember the exciting times when Prof Dr. Altchek started to discuss the possibility of uterine transplant with Swedish professor Dr. Mats Brännström.

After the first uterine transplant was performed in Sweden, the United States was next, with a successful uterine transplant in 2016. To date, only one Swedish and one U.S. center have previously published findings of livebirths from transplanted uteri [46, 47]. Now uterine transplantation centers exist worldwide, offering hopes to women who aren't otherwise able to carry a pregnancy.

8 Conclusions

Hormonal therapy for gender dysphoria and for congenital anomalies is a very complex subject, with particular features for each condition but also with some common general principles. In conditions where a lack of a hormone is known, addition of that hormone to the regimen makes sense; the devil, as always, would be in the details. Yes, it is simple and logical to administer testosterone when one lacks 5-alpha-reductase or to administer the final product of an enzymatic pathway when that particular enzyme is missing, but there are so many clinical situations that one has to tailor the treatments accordingly.

Hormones may be given for initiation of puberty or development of sexual characteristics, or they may be given for reaching a state of "congruent" with the desired gender, for contraception or as a replacement therapy, among other uses. In doing so, treatments in general try to imitate the physiologic ways; therefore, many times hormonal treatment is started with small doses, and in some cases, other hormones are added to the therapy with the purpose of preventing unwanted side effects.

Among all the organs affected by hormonal treatments, uterus (with its lining, the endometrium) is one of the most remarkable in its responses. In a physiologic situation, the endometrium will react differently to estrogen and progesterone cyclic changes, showing a different morphology each day of the menstrual cycle. Similarly, the endometrium will react to hormones administered for a plethora of reasons, from contraceptives, ovarian stimulation for infertility, menopausal replacement treatment, treatments of benign or malignant (e.g., breast cancer) tumors, and the patterns of the responses will be extremely diverse, making interpretation of biopsies very challenging.

Last but not least, the psychological aspects of all medical conditions requiring hormonal treatment are worth mentioning. Treating these patients is a long-term commitment, requiring team work which involves practitioners from different fields (general practitioners, endocrinologists, pediatricians, gynecologists, surgeons, radiologists, oncologists, etc.) as well as patient support groups. Aside from the correct diagnosis and multifaceted treatment, doctors should also be aware of the anxiety and depression these human beings experience and should always offer counseling and support.

References

1. Martine Rothblatt. The apartheid of sex.
2. American Psychiatric Association. Diagnostic and statistical manual of mental disorders. 5th ed. Arlington, VA: American Psychiatric Association; 2013. p. 451–9.
3. Frisén L, Söder O, Rydelius PA. Dramatic increase of gender dysphoria in youth. Läkartidningen. 2017.
4. Cartaya J, Lopez X. Gender dysphoria in youth: a review of recent literature. Curr Opin Endocrinol Diabetes Obes. 2018;25(1):44–8.
5. Aitken M, Steensma TD, Blanchard R, et al. Evidence for an altered sex ratio in clinic-referred adolescents with gender dysphoria. J Sex Med. 2015;12:756–63.
6. Streed CG Jr, McCarthy EP, Haas JS. Association between gender minority status and self-reported physical and mental health in the United States. JAMA Intern Med. 2017;177:1210–2.
7. Klein DA, Paradise SL, Goodwin ET. Caring for transgender and gender-diverse persons: what clinicians should know. Am Fam Physician. 2018;98(11):645–53.
8. WPATH. Clarification on medical necessity of treatment, sex reassignment, and insurance coverage for transgender and transsexual people worldwide [Internet]. http://www.wpath.org/site_page.cfm?pk_association_webpage_menu=1352&pk_association_webpage=3947
9. Coleman E, Bockting W, Botzer M, Cohen-Kettenis P, DeCuypere G, Feldman J, et al. Standards of care for the health of transsexual, transgender, and gender-nonconforming people, version 7. Int J Transgenderism. 2012;13(4):165–232.
10. Joint R, Chen ZE, Cameron S. Breast and reproductive cancers in the transgender population: a systematic review [published online ahead of print April 28, 2018]. BJOG. 2018;125:1505. https://doi.org/10.1111/1471-0528.15258.
11. Maraka S, Singh Ospina N, Rodriguez-Gutierrez R, et al. Sex steroids and cardiovascular outcomes in transgender individuals: a systematic review and meta-analysis. J Clin Endocrinol Metab. 2017;102(11):3914–23.
12. Singh-Ospina N, Maraka S, Rodriguez-Gutierrez R, et al. Effect of sex steroids on the bone health of transgender individuals: a systematic review and meta-analysis. J Clin Endocrinol Metab. 2017;102(11):3904–13.
13. Meriggiola MC, Gava G. Endocrine care of transpeople part I. A review of cross-sex hormonal treatments, outcomes and adverse effects in transmen. Clin Endocrinol. 2015;83(5):597–606.
14. Weinand JD, Safer JD. Hormone therapy in transgender adults is safe with provider supervision; a review of hormone therapy sequelae for transgender individuals. J Clin Transl Endocrinol. 2015;2(2):55–60.
15. Deutsch MB. Guidelines for the primary and gender-affirming care of transgender and gender nonbinary people. 2nd ed. 2016. http://transhealth.ucsf.edu/protocols. Accessed 5 July 2018.
16. Endocrine Society Updates Guidelines on Transgender Medical Care. Veronica Hackenthal. 2017. www.medscape.com

17. Hembree WC, Cohen-Kettenis PT, Gooren L, et al. Endocrine treatment of gender-dysphoric/gender-incongruent persons: an Endocrine. Society clinical practice guideline [published correction appears in J Clin Endocrinol Metab. 2018;103(2):699]. J Clin Endocrinol Metab. 2017;102(11):3869–903.
18. Moore E, Wisniewski A, Dobs A. Endocrine treatment of transsexual people: a review of treatment regimens, outcomes, and adverse effects. J Clin Endocrinol Metab. 2003;88(8):3467–73.
19. Brown GR, Jones KT. Incidence of breast cancer in a cohort of 5,135 transgender veterans. Breast Cancer Res Treat. 2015;149(1):191–8.
20. Gooren L, Morgentaler A. Prostate cancer incidence in orchidectomised male-to-female transsexual persons treated with oestrogens. Andrologia. 2014;46(10):1156–60.
21. Turo R, Jallad S, Prescott S, Cross WR. Metastatic prostate cancer in transsexual diagnosed after three decades of estrogen therapy. Can Urol Assoc J. 2013;7(7–8):E544–6.
22. Spratt DI, Stewart II, Savage C, et al. Subcutaneous injection of testosterone is an effective and preferred alternative to intramuscular injection: demonstration in female-to-male transgender patients. J Clin Endocrinol Metab. 2017;102:2349–55.
23. Costa LBF, Rosa-E-Silva ACJS, Medeiros SF, Nacul AP, Carvalho BR, Benetti-Pinto CL, Yela DA, Maciel GAR, Soares Júnior JM, Maranhão TMO. Recommendations for the use of testosterone in male transgender. Rev Bras Ginecol Obstet. 2018;40(5):275–80.
24. Wierckx K, Mueller S, Weyers S, Van Caenegem E, Roef G, Heylens G, et al. Long-term evaluation of cross-sex hormone treatment in transsexual persons. J Sex Med. 2012;9(10):2641–51.
25. Urban RR, Teng NNH, Kapp DS. Gynecologic malignancies in female-to-male transgender patients: the need of original gender surveillance. Am J Obstet Gynecol. 2011;204(5):e9–12.
26. Grynberg M, Fanchin R, Dubost G, Colau J-C, Brémont-Weil C, Frydman R, et al. Histology of genital tract and breast tissue after long-term testosterone administration in a female-to-male transsexual population. Reprod Biomed Online. 2010;20(4):553–8.
27. Perrone AM, Cerpolini S, Maria Salfi NC, Ceccarelli C, De Giorgi LB, Formelli G, et al. Effect of long-term testosterone administration on the endometrium of female-to-male (FtM) transsexuals. J Sex Med. 2009;6(11):3193–200.
28. Dizon DS, Tejada-Berges T, Koelliker S, Steinhoff M, Granai CO. Ovarian cancer associated with testosterone supplementation in a female-to-male transsexual patient. Gynecol Obstet Investig. 2006;62(4):226–8.
29. Hage JJ, Dekker JJ, Karim RB, Verheijen RH, Bloemena E. Ovarian cancer in female-to-male transsexuals: report of two cases. Gynecol Oncol. 2000;76(3):413–5.
30. Futterweit W, Deligdisch L. Histopathological effects of exogenously administered testosterone in 19 female to male transsexuals. J Clin Endocrinol Metab. 1986;62(1):16–21.
31. Futterweit W, Deligdisch L. Effects of androgens on the ovary. Fertil Steril. 1986;46(2):343–5.
32. Wierckx K, Elaut E, Declercq E, Heylens G, De Cuypere G, Taes Y, et al. Prevalence of cardiovascular disease and cancer during cross-sex hormone therapy in a large cohort of trans persons: a case-control study. Eur J Endocrinol. 2013;169(4):471–8.
33. American Fertility Society. The American Fertility Society classifications of adnexal adhesions, distal tubal occlusion, tubal occlusion secondary to tubal ligation, tubal pregnancies, Müllerian anomalies and intrauterine adhesions. Fertil Steril. 1988;49:944–55.
34. Chandler TM, Machan LS, Cooperberg PL, Harris AC, Chang SD. Müllerian duct anomalies: from diagnosis to intervention. Pictorial review. Brit J Radiol. 2009;82:1034–42.
35. Grimbizis GF, Campo R, Gordts S, Brucker S, Gergolet M, Tanos V, et al. Clinical approach for the classification of congenital uterine malformations. Gynecol Surg. 2012;9:119–29.
36. Grimbizis GF, Gordts S, Spiezio Sardo A, Brucker S, De Angelis C, Gergolet M, et al. The ESHRE/ESGE consensus on the classification of female genital tract congenital anomalies. Hum Reprod. 2013;28:2032–44.
37. Acién P, Acién M. Diagnostic imaging and cataloguing of female genital malformations. Insights Imaging. 2016;7(5):713–26.
38. Witchel SF. Disorders of sex development. Best Pract Res Clin Obstet Gynaecol. 2018;48:90–102.

39. Lee PA, Nordenström A, Houk CP, et al. Global disorders of sex development update since 2006: perceptions, approach and care. Horm Res Paediatr. 2016;85:158–80.
40. Hughes IA, Nihoul-Fékété C, Thomas B, et al. Consequences of the ESPE/LWPES guidelines for diagnosis and treatment of disorders of sex development. Best Pract Res Clin Endocrinol Metab. 2007;21:351–65.
41. Chen MJ, McCann-Crosby B, Gunn S, et al. Fluidity models in ancient Greece and current practices of sex assignment. Semin Perinatol. 2017;41:206–13.
42. Patel V, Casey RK, Gomez-Lobo V. Timing of gonadectomy in patients with complete androgen insensitivity syndrome-current recommendations and future directions. J Pediatr Adolesc Gynecol. 2016;29:320–5.
43. Laurian L, Finkelstein JO, Soferman N, Loewenthal M, Deligdisch L. Testicular feminization syndrome. Isr J Med Sci. 1971;7(5):668–73.
44. Becker D, Wain LM, Chong YH, Gosai SJ, Henderson NK, Milburn J, Stott V, Wheeler BJ. Topical dihydrotestosterone to treat micropenis secondary to partial androgen insensitivity syndrome (PAIS) before, during, and after puberty—a case series. J Pediatr Endocrinol Metab. 2016;29(2):173–7.
45. Altchek A, Deligdisch L. Pediatric adolescent and young adult gynecology: Blackwell Publishing; 2009.
46. Brännström M, Johannesson L, Bokström H, et al. Livebirth after uterus transplantation. Lancet. 2015;385:607–16.
47. Testa G, McKenna GJ, Gunby RT Jr, et al. First live birth after uterus transplantation in the United States. Am Transplant. 2018;18:1270–4.

Hormone Therapy Effects on the Uterus

Liane Deligdisch-Schor

1 General Considerations

The uterine tissue is exquisitely sensitive to hormonal influences, being able to translate them into functional and structural changes with promptitude and versatility. The complex interplay mediated by finely tuned feedback mechanisms between pituitary gland and gonadal functions, functionally related to the central nervous system, reaches its target in the uterine tissue securing the reproductive role of the uterus. Normal reproduction is based on the cyclic changes taking place in the entire female genital system and especially in the inner lining of the uterus, the endometrium. The programming of events in the endometrium, a highly differentiated and diversified tissue (glands, stroma, blood vessels), is regulated by the presence of receptors, essential to the transfers and translocation of the hormones secreted into the blood stream, and their translation into structural changes at the target tissue.

The most commonly involved gonad-secreted hormones are steroid hormones, estrogens and progesterone, bound to receptors, forming hormone-receptor complexes. The activated steroid receptor functions as a transcription factor modulating the synthesis of specific mRNA, responsible for the cellular action of the hormone. The receptor-bound hormone is transported into the cellular compartments, from replenishment in the cytoplasm to "shuttling" into nuclear chromatin-bound complexes which dispatch it to organelles by recruiting cell-specific signal-modifying proteins resulting in effects on cells such as proliferation, secretion, and apoptosis in normal cycles [1].

L. Deligdisch-Schor (✉)
Professor Emeritus, Department of Pathology, The Icahn School of Medicine at Mount Sinai, New York, NY, USA

Department of Obstetrics-Gynecology and Reproductive Science, The Icahn School of Medicine at Mount Sinai, New York, NY, USA

L. Deligdisch-Schor, A. Mareş Miceli (eds.), *Hormonal Pathology of the Uterus*, Advances in Experimental Medicine and Biology 1242,
https://doi.org/10.1007/978-3-030-38474-6_8

The biologic activity of the steroid hormones is maintained only while the nuclear site is occupied by the hormone-receptor complex, thus duration of exposure, as well as concentration are related to effect. The absence or decrease of hormones results eventually in atrophic changes; the excess of hormones may produce irregular patterns of proliferation, hyperplasia, and neoplasia. Clinically, abnormal hormonal stimulation may be associated with infertility, abnormal vaginal bleeding (prolonged, irregular or reduced), often associated with benign lesions such as leiomyomas, adenomyosis, endometrial polyps, and uterine neoplasia, as well as a host of systemic disorders such as those encountered in peri- and post-menopausal syndromes.

Hormone therapy is used to counteract the deleterious effects of "natural", noniatrogenic, abnormal hormonal function. Hormone therapy is now widely prescribed, being used by millions of women all over the world. It seems that actually most women would use at least some hormone therapy at some point of their life. Adolescents and young women use oral contraceptives, sometime also prescribed during the perimenopausal years. Hormones are prescribed for irregular vaginal bleeding, uterine enlargement due to leiomyoma and adenomyosis, for symptoms due to hormone deprivation as in menopause or premature ovarian failure. Hormone therapy is used for infertility associated in numerous cases with hormonal inadequacy and reproductive technology includes ovulation stimulation by hormones. Postmenopausal symptoms are widely treated with hormones despite controversial data on their safety and efficiency; the regimens are shifting being almost permanently subjects for change. Hormone therapy is used for the adjuvant treatment of breast and uterine cancer, most frequently for reversal of endometrial hyperplasia. Tamoxifen, successfully used in breast cancer, is sometime associated with endometrial neoplasms, polyps, and endometrial carcinoma. Hormone therapy is also used for treatment of congenital abnormal sexual development and of gender dysphoria.

Hormone therapy elicits important changes in the physiopathology and structure of uterine tissues. These changes are difficult to be adequately and reliably described in textbooks because of the diversity of the histological, histochemical, and immunohistological patterns resulting from permanently changing therapeutic regimens, multiple and often controversial concepts, changing statistical data and identification of new cellular markers.

Uterine biopsies, mostly endometrial biopsies obtained by D&C or endometrial aspirates routinely used during or after hormone therapy in order to evaluate the effects on the endometrial tissue and occasionally on the myometrium and other pelvic structures, are often difficult to interpret. Confusion with premalignant and frankly neoplastic tissues, for example in estrogen-induced glandular hyperplasia with stromal breakdown, may occur. Underdiagnosis of an iatrogenically modified malignant tissue, such as decidualized stroma and secretory glands in endometrial neoplasm under progestin hormonal therapy, can be dangerously misleading.

The microscopic analysis of histologic changes in the uterine, especially endometrial tissue submitted to hormonal therapeutic manipulations, reveals the response or lack thereof to the administered, mostly, steroid hormones which is closely related to the abundance and distribution pattern of receptors and other significant proteins. This is detectable by immunohistologic markers used in special stains of the sectioned tissue; molecular biology research demonstrates a permanent renewal of these markers.

It therefore appears that the uterus, an organ composed of tissues highly sensitive and receptive to hormones due to the abundance of receptors, is capable of profound and diverse structural changes with a wide variety of patterns on microscopic examination, resulting from physiological and pathological hormonal influences. The interpretation of these patterns becomes more complex and difficult as the administration of hormones is permanently changing regimens and dosages, and is modified by new products and new concepts.

The following histopathologic descriptions are describing the relevant changes of the uterus, especially of the endometrium, consistent with diagnostic categories, in most commonly used hormonal therapies.

2 Iatrogenic Hormonal Effects on the Uterus

2.1 Hormonal Contraceptive Therapy

The most commonly, effectively used contraceptive method is based on hormonal suppression of ovulation and increase of cervical mucus density. The first "pill" was marketed and approved for use in the United States in the early 1960s with the name of ENOVID. It was composed of both estrogen (ethynyl estradiol) and progesterone/progestin. Hormonal contraception was first administered sequentially as an attempt to imitate the natural menstrual cycle, first estrogen then progesterone. This method however turned out to be relatively unsafe, with occasional failures to prevent pregnancy, irregular vaginal bleeding, and some cases of endometrial hyperplasia and neoplasia [2, 3]. In 1970, sequential hormone contraception was suspended in the United States. Since then, the most commonly administered "pill" is the combined estrogen-progesterone and more recently the progesterone-only pill. The most common hormonal contraception is the oral contraception (OC). Hormonal contraception also includes subcutaneous "patches" implants, intravaginal rings, intrauterine devices, and injections, all based on long-lasting release of steroid hormones, mainly progesterone.

The ovulation suppression is based on the negative feedback of estrogen and progesterone on the gonadotropin-releasing hormone (GnRH) secreted by the anterior pituitary lobe under hypothalamic stimulation, with decrease of follicle-stimulating and luteinizing hormones (FSH and LH), resulting in follicle development inhibition and preventing the mid-cycle surge of LH with absent ovulation. Cervical mucus becomes less permeable for sperm, mostly due to the progesterone effect.

Combined OC are also used for noncontraceptive purposes, and also for the treatment of polycystic ovarian syndrome, hirsutism, menstrual disorders, and menorrhagia. The effect of hormonal contraceptives on the endometrium is related to dosage and potency of the hormones. High-dose high-potency OC, not any more used in the United States in recent years, produces marked stromal hyperplasia with decidual reaction, smooth muscle hyperplasia suggestive of neoplasia (pseudosarcoma), and glandular atrophy of the endometrial tissue (Fig. 1). Currently used regimens containing lower doses and lower potency produce an arrest of proliferation in the first cycles with straight or slightly coiled glands lined by immature epithelial cells with nuclei showing an evenly distributed chromatin network. The thick nuclear membrane, coarse chromatin clumps, and mitotic activity seen in natural cycling proliferative endometrium, are absent. The cytoplasm contains randomly distributed vacuoles, and the apical border, unlike that of natural secretory endometrium, is smooth and well defined (Fig. 2).

The endometrial microscopic appearance on biopsies from women taking hormonal contraceptives display a variety of changes related to the effect of the hormones taken, their strength, dosage, duration of treatment (Table 1). The age of the patient, metabolic disturbances such as obesity or diabetes, hyperestrogenic conditions like ovarian hyperthecosis, polycystic syndrome, endometriosis may influence the response to hormonal contraception. Locally in the uterine tissue, the amount and distribution of receptors is related to the changes of tissue architectural structure and of the individual cells.

The predominant effect of the combined OC pill on the endometrial target tissue is that of progesterone featuring an appearance somehow resembling the secretory postovulatory endometrium, however, with major differences. The normal, natural

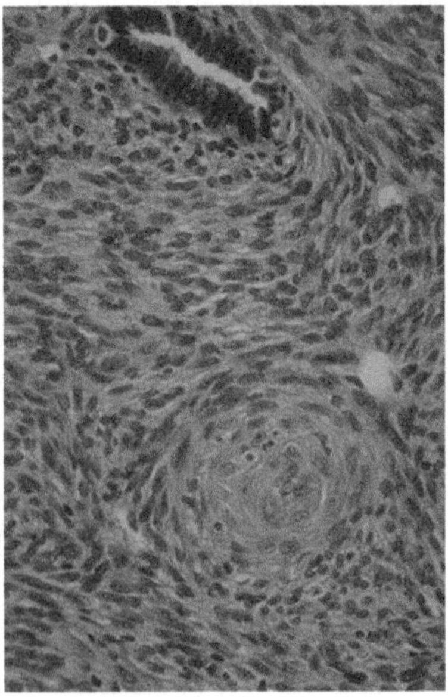

Fig. 1 Effect of high-potency OC: endometrial stromal and smooth muscle hyperplasia (pseudosarcoma), H&E ×100

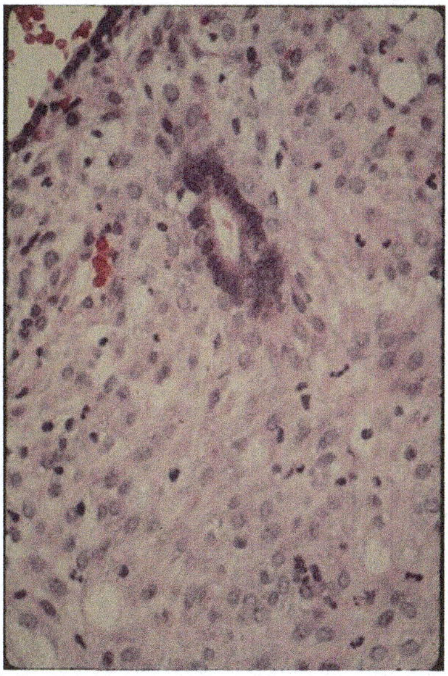

Fig. 2 OC effect on endometrium: inactive gland lined by immature cuboidal epithelial cells with scant abortive secretion in lumen and stromal decidual reaction with scattered leukocytes. H&E ×100

Table 1 Endometrial histology in oral contraceptive therapy

Predominant stroma over glands volume	
Glands	Arrest of epithelial proliferation
	Absent or abortive secretion
	Linear apical cell border
Stroma	Early edema
	Decidual reaction/ pseudopregnancy decidua
	Scattered leukocytes
Blood vessels	Absent spiral arterioles
	Venous sinusoidal dilation
Inactive or atrophic endometrium in prolonged OC therapy	

proportion of endometrial glandular versus stromal tissue is about 50/50%. With the predominantly progestational effect of hormonal contraceptives, the stroma becomes voluminous, and the glandular compartment is markedly reduced to an extent depending on the duration of the hormone administration (Fig. 3). The stroma is first edematous then gradually becomes decidualized with plump pavement-like cells with round nuclei and an abundant cytoplasm loaded with glucose, polymucosaccharides, proteins, and other nutrients destined for a possibly implanting blastocyst, as in natural endometrial cycles. However, the glands which are secretory in normal postovulatory cycles, with first subnuclear then supranuclear glycogen vacuoles, or as in later days of the cycle, "sawmill"-shaped with abundant secretion in the lumen, do not show these features with OC therapy: They appear rather inactive,

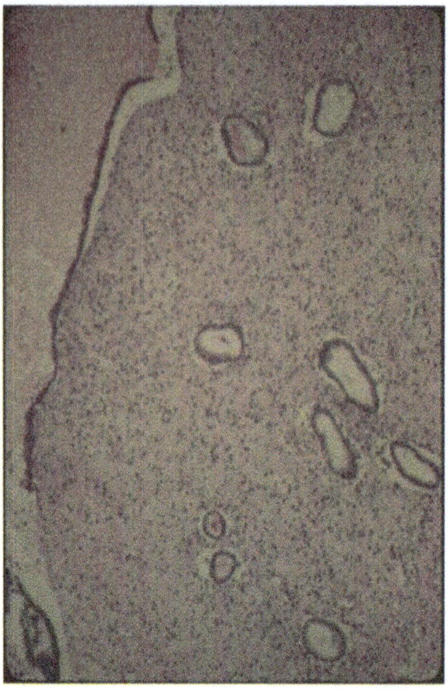

Fig. 3 OC effect on endometrium: stromal hyperplasia and rarefied inactive to atrophic glands. H&E ×40

small, tubular, straight, and lined by cuboidal or flat epithelial cells, with a straight luminal border and occasional droplets of secretion in their lumen (abortive secretion as in Fig. 2).

The blood vessels which in natural, functional cycles become thickened and coiled ("spiral arterioles") presenting an increased surface, therefore more chances for implantation for a possible fertilized ovum whose trophoblast is "searching" for spiral arterioles containing maternal blood, are thin and straight with OC therapy. Some blood vessels are abnormally dilated, containing blood clots. Superficial dilated venules and scattered lymphoid and polymorphonuclear leukocytes are present. Angiectasis and thrombosis are associated with breakthrough bleeding occurring sometime under progesterone-dominated contraceptive regimen.

The histologic appearance of the endometrium is not consistent with any physiological phase of the "dating" system used by pathologists to determine the adequacy of endometrial cyclic development for gestational purposes (Figs. 2 and 3). The endometrium treated with hormonal contraceptives is profoundly inadequate for implantation of a fertilized ovum, i.e., blastocyst; therefore, even if ovulation and fertilization took place, the decidualized endometrium, especially its compact surface will not permit implantation as it mimics pregnancy changes (pseudopregnancy endometrium). An already pregnant uterus cannot become pregnant! Experienced gynecologic pathologists recognize the "contraceptive endometrium" on the discrepancy between edematous (early-stage therapy) then decidualized (pseudogestational) and eventually thinned endometrial stroma and the inactive nonsecretory glands as well as the absence of spiral arterioles. The presence in the endometrial stroma of scattered leukocytes among decidual cells is an uncharacteristic finding for natural cycles in which numerous leukocytes infiltrate the stroma shortly before the apoptotic changes of endometrial glandular epithelium and stroma during menstrual shedding. Prolonged use of hormonal contraceptive therapy may elicit a gradual atrophy of endometrial glands and thinning of the endometrial stroma with reduced decidual change. Also described in women taking OC is endocervical microglandular hyperplasia (Fig. 4) sometime with squamous metaplasia, similar to that seen in pregnancy.

The histologic patterns seen in endometrial biopsies from women receiving OC are unlike any "natural" noniatrogenic endometrial pattern, normal or pathologic. The combination of inactive glands, abortive secretion, and decidual stroma with thin blood vessels is characteristic of only OC therapy.

Progesterone receptor modulators (PRM), such as mifepristone, are used for contraception as well. Their effect on the endometrium appears to be mixed secretory, proliferative, and inactive glands with some cystic dilation [4]. The use of PRM as contraceptives is debatable and histological studies are limited; no malignant developments have been reported with this therapy.

2.2 *Hormonal Therapy for Infertility*

A large proportion of infertility cases are related to hormonal anomalies eliciting premature ovarian failure, anovulatory cycles, and/or amenorrhea. The most commonly employed method to "reactivate" the endometrial cyclic changes preparing the maternal tissue to host an implanting blastocyst is to stimulate the ovary to both ovulate and secrete steroid hormones that will elicit structural changes in the uterine

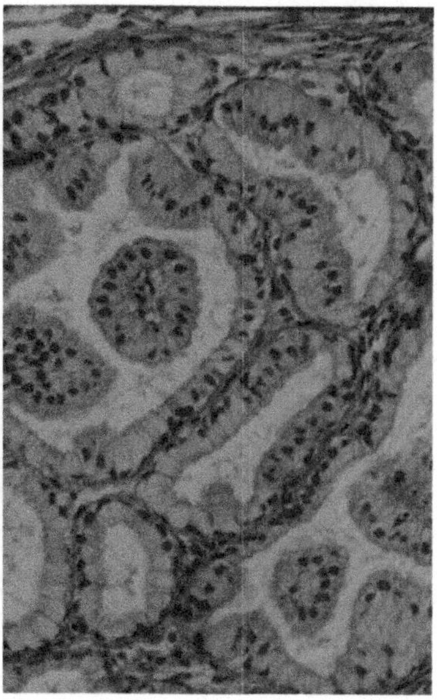

Fig. 4 Effect of OC: Endocervical gland hyperplasia. H&E ×100

target tissues, mainly the endometrium, and also in the myometrial tissue. The hormones that stimulate the ovary are chiefly gonadotropin-releasing hormones (GnRH) and their agonists, follicle-stimulating hormone (FSH), and luteinizing hormone (LH), to be secreted by the anterior lobe of the pituitary gland. Ovarian stimulation inhibits the negative feedback at the level of the thalamus and therefore stimulates the secretion of GnRH re-establishing the cyclic fertility-promoting hormonal activities of the uterus [1]. The response of the target tissues is variable but improves constantly, and successful pregnancies obtained with ovulation stimulation are numerous (see Chapter 2). Clomiphene citrate, a SERM, is frequently used, sometimes with associated steroid hormones. Multiple gestations are more common due to multiple ovulation as an ovarian stimulation effect; fortunately, overstimulation syndrome with occasional serious deleterious consequences, such as ovarian infarct and peritonitis, are presently very rare (Fig. 5).

The purpose of ovarian stimulation is the establishment of regular cyclic ovulation following normal follicle maturation and timely release of the ovule(s) at ovulation. The uterine tissues are prepared to serve as hosts to the implanting conceptus by modulating functions and structures adequately under the influences of estrogen and progesterone secreted cyclically by granulosa cells in the maturing, stimulated follicle and by the corpus luteum promptly after ovulation. The uterine target tissues are expected to respond adequately by normal proliferation and secretion, as in spontaneous normal cycles. Histologic studies of endometrial D&C tissue obtained in cases of subsequent failures concluded that no single finding seemed to be relevant for spontaneous pregnancy termination occurring in pregnancies which develop after iatrogenic ovulation stimulation [5]. The secretory changes in glands were observed to lag behind the secretory changes in the stroma, with subnuclear and supranuclear vacuoles in the glandular epithelium concomitant with decidual stro-

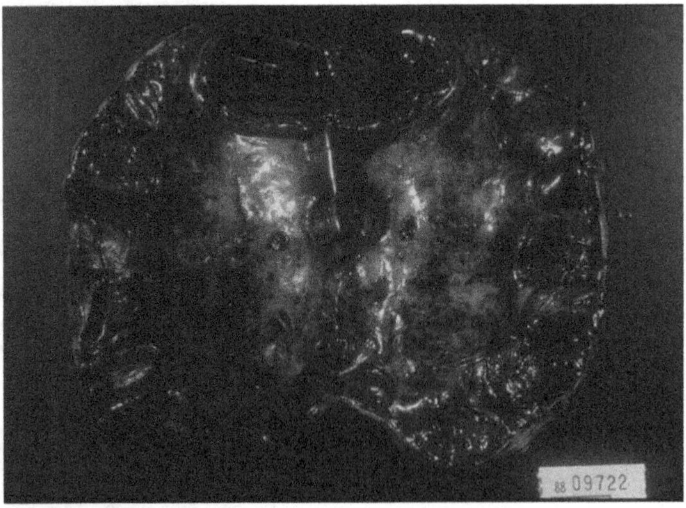

Fig. 5 Infarcted ovary due to iatrogenic hyperstimulation

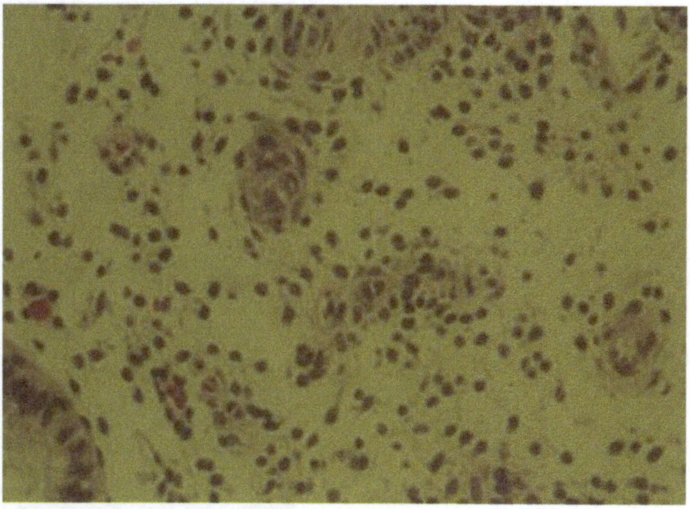

Fig. 6 Effect of ovulation stimulation: secretory endometrium with spiral arterioles surrounded by decidual reaction consistent with day 22–23. H&E ×40

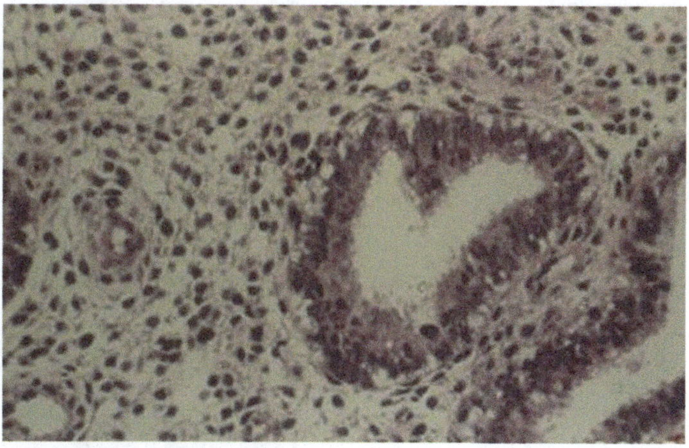

Fig. 7 Same endometrial biopsy: secretory glands with sub- and supranuclear vacuoles consistent with day 16–17. H&E ×100

mal reaction and spiral arterioles (Figs. 6 and 7). Mild inflammatory infiltrates can be present during early gestation possibly representing autoimmune endometritis [6].

An unusual serious complication occurred leading to a first trimester abortion in a patient after ovarian stimulation. The patient had a history of polycystic ovarian disease and endometrial glandular hyperplasia, and was treated with hormonal ovulation stimulation that resulted in a triplet gestation. She aborted at 9 weeks

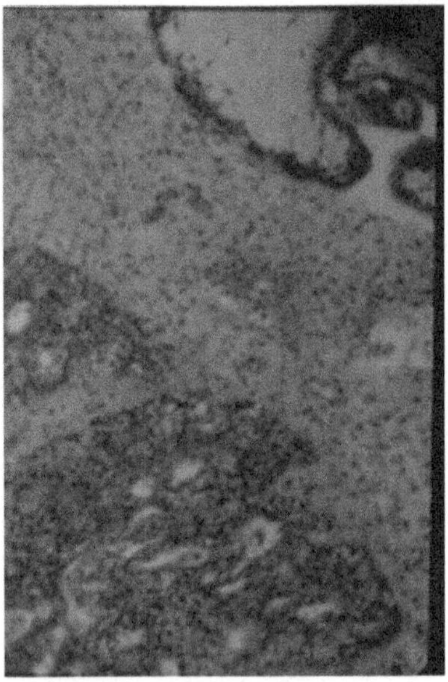

Fig. 8 Unusual "bedfellows" in endometrial biopsy: gestational and neoplastic changes of endometrium in aborted triplet pregnancy after ovulation stimulation of patient with previous polycystic ovarian disease and endometrial glandular hyperplasia. Chorionic villi (upper right corner), decidua, adenocarcinoma (lower left corner). H&E ×40

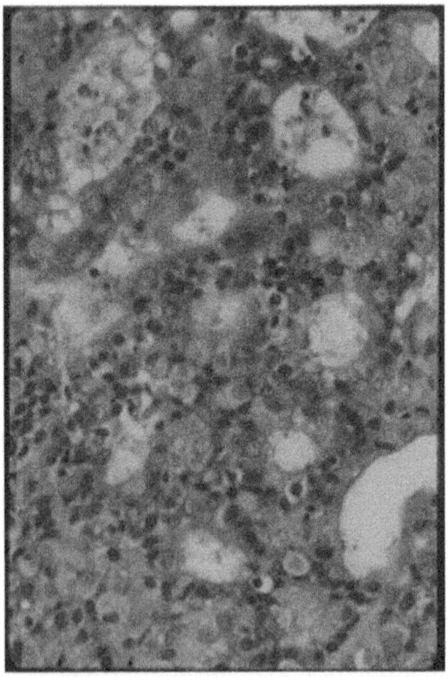

Fig. 9 Same endometrial biopsy: adenocarcinoma, endometrioid type with secretory features. H&E ×100

gestation. The histologic examination of the endometrial curettings revealed an endometrial adenocarcinoma in addition to the products of conception (chorionic villi) and endometrial stromal decidualization (Figs. 8 and 9). The malignant tumor probably developed in the hyperplastic endometrium associated with polycystic ovarian disease, most likely prior to the pregnancy. The association of malignant and gestational endometrial changes is very rare; it was suggested that it could be prevented by a previously inserted progestin intrauterine device [7].

2.3 *Effects of Hormone Therapy on Benign Uterine Lesions*

2.3.1 Leiomyomas

Leiomyomas are the most common benign tumors of the uterus, originating in the smooth muscle and in the vascular wall of the uterus. They form nodular masses located under the endometrium (submucosal), under the serosa (subserosal), in the myometrial wall (intramural), often reaching large dimensions. Once symptomatic due to sensations of heaviness, compression of neighboring organs such as urinary bladder or rectum, or protruding into the endometrial cavity causing abnormal vaginal bleeding by stretching the endometrium and increasing its surface, thus causing abundant menstrual shedding, surgery becomes the most indicated therapeutic choice.

Hormone therapy, however, is an alternative or a therapeutic adjuvant as uterine leiomyomas are strongly related to estrogenic influence, developing most commonly during the reproductive age and gradually shrinking after menopause. Gonadotropic-releasing hormone (GnRH) analogues have been used to reduce the size of leiomyomata by inducing an iatrogenic reversible menopause with up to 70% shrinking of their volume over a relatively short period of time. This therapy usually does not exceed 2–3 months as the size reduction generally takes place during this time, and side effects of an early menopause have to be minimized.

The mechanism of shrinking has been analyzed by histopathologic examination of the lesions in consecutive phases of treatment as compared to untreated (control) leiomyomas [8]. The central areas of the nodules display edema and hydropic degeneration that appears as "geographic" areas (Fig. 10) followed by collagen fiber

Fig. 10 Effect of 1-month Lupron therapy on leiomyoma: central edema, peripheral fibrosis. H&E ×25

proliferation and hyaline degeneration (Fig. 11). Necrosis of myometrial tissue surrounded by areas of hypercellularity was also present, with focal mild to moderate atypia. Lymphoid cell aggregates were observed in the treated cased and absent in the control. The interface between the myomatous nodule and the surrounding myometrium appeared blurred, with obliteration of the cleavage plan (Fig. 12a)—a change that may result in a more difficult surgical enucleation of the shrunken nodule. The edematous, hydropic, and necrotic areas become hyalinized forming confluent retracted scar-like plaques (Fig. 12b).

These histologic features when present in subsequent myomectomy or hysterectomy specimens are consistent with previous GnRH (Lupron) therapy resulting in smaller tumor masses at the time of surgery. The rather spectacular effect of size reduction with GnRH analogue therapy over a short period of time in most cases demonstrates the ability of the myometrial tissue to respond promptly to hormonal influences, due to hormone receptors present in the myometrial tissue. Therapy with GnRH analogues induces an iatrogenic menopause by suppressing the estrogenic stimulation as a result of decreased gonadotropin secretion. This response represents an accelerated version of the physiological postmenopausal shrinking over a longer period of time when both myomas and myometrium become smaller and eventually atrophic due to absent hormonal stimulation. Myomatous nodules in normally atrophic postmenopausal uteri are hyalinized and often calcified. Postmenopausal estrogenic stimulation may result in enlargement of myomatous uteri. Progesterone applied in intrauterine devices (IUD) or given as a contraceptive does not really reduce leiomyomas, but its effect on the endometrium is to stop proliferation and induce secretory changes, decidual reaction and eventually atrophy, and to stop the vaginal bleeding. On myomectomy and hysterectomy specimens,

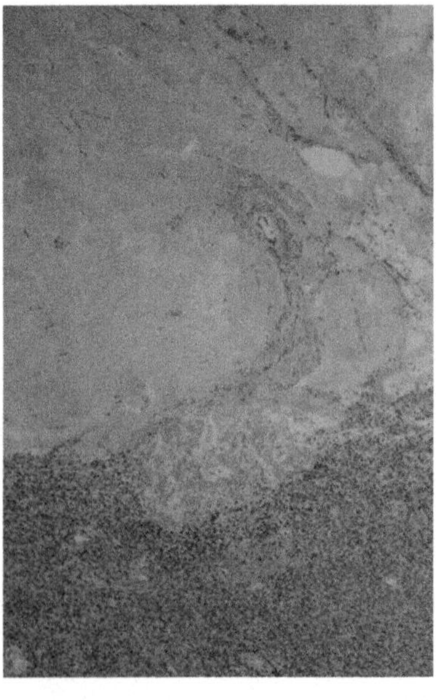

Fig. 11 Effect of 3-months Lupron therapy on leiomyoma: hyalinized retracted scar. H&E ×25

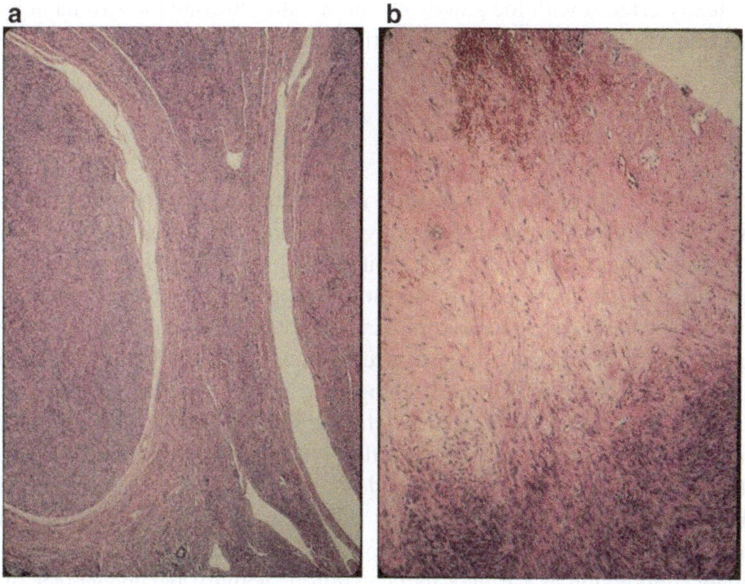

Fig. 12 (**a**) Untreated leiomyoma: cleavage plan at the myoma–myometrial interface. (**b**) Effect of Lupron therapy on leiomyoma: hyalinized zone of retraction obstructing cleavage plan from surrounding myometrium. H&E ×25

it has been shown that previous progesterone therapy elicited softening of the nodules, microscopically mild to moderate cellular atypia and occasional necrosis.

Ulipristol acetate aims also to shrink myomas in a way similar to GnRH, but its efficiency is not proven as yet [9].

Progesterone-receptor modulators (PRM) were evaluated in the management of endometriosis, adenomyosis, and leiomyomata due to their interaction with the progesterone receptor to inhibit or stimulate a downstream hormonal response. Their effect on endometrial histology included inactive or normal-appearing cyclic endometrium, discrepancy between glandular and stromal development, coexistent proliferative and secretory features, and occasional cystically dilated glands lined by a mixed mitotically active proliferative and a secretory endometrium; hyperplastic and neoplastic changes of the endometrium were not reported [4].

2.3.2 Adenomyosis

Adenomyosis is the presence of endometrial tissue (glands, stroma, and blood vessels) in the myometrium, which are also stimulated by estrogens and progesterone, therefore responsive to hormone therapy in a similar way as leiomyomas. With GnRH therapy and/or progesterone, there is shrinking of the affected regions in the uterus. Microscopically, the islands of endometrial tissue surrounded by myometrium are gradually effaced with the glands becoming atrophic and the stroma dense and fibrotic, in a manner similar to the involution taking place after menopause.

2.3.3 Endometrial Polyps

These mostly benign endometrial lesions are a frequent cause of abnormal vaginal bleeding at any age but most commonly peri- and post-menopausal. Thickened blood vessels are central to a stalk surrounded by endometrial stroma and glands that are often cystic, both poor in hormone receptors, therefore maintaining the same structure throughout the menstrual cycle, occasionally causing intermenstrual vaginal bleeding. Hormonal contraceptive therapy does not elicit much change in the glands of the polyp which are keeping their mostly inactive appearance; their stroma is composed of fibroblasts and rich in collagen fibers. Postmenopausal polyps may be large due to cystic glandular dilation causing postmenopausal bleeding for which surgical removal is recommended. Hormone therapy is used in endometrial hyperplasia with polypoid growth (hyperplastic polyps) which is usually responsive to progesterone. The effects on the endometrium are evident as dose-dependent suppression of estrogen-induced mitotic activity and appearance of glandular secretion and stromal decidual reaction.

3 Hormone Replacement Therapy Effects on Uterus

With the prolongation of life expectancy, the postmenopausal period may last one-third or more of a woman's lifetime. Postmenopausal morbidity is chiefly caused by the gradual decrease followed by the absence of natural estrogen secretion due to regressing ovarian function. Among the most common symptoms are hot flashes, urogenital atrophy, insomnia, anxiety, osteoporosis, hyperlipidemia that may lead to threatening cardiovascular and cerebrovascular morbidity. Estrogens and estrogen derivatives were used for decades in the last century. In the 1970s, however it became clear that using estrogens alone or estrogen/progesterone sequentially, as an imitation of natural cyclic activity, during the reproductive years, is associated with a risk for endometrial hyperplasia and neoplasia [10, 11]. Since then, sequential hormone replacement therapy (HRT) was replaced with combined HRT for women who kept their uterus. This therapy has been administered on a large scale (to ~38% of women in the United States), despite multiple controversial opinions, and is permanently changing [12–14].

The estrogen/progesterone HRT regimens are different from those used for oral contraceptives, mainly because of the significantly lower dosages and the different hormonal types used. HRT is the object of numerous controversial opinions. The results of the largest randomized clinical trial of HRT by the Women Health Initiative (WHI) published in 2002 were surprising by showing an increase of postmenopausal morbidity (pulmonary emboli, coronary heart disease, stroke, breast cancer), also suggesting deleterious effects from the associated progesterone [13]. This was contested by subsequent meta-analysis based on the evaluation of the patients age. It was concluded that HRT initiated early after menopause, in younger patients, and lasting not more than 5 years is rather beneficial, as older patients may have had cardiovascular disorders that are worsening, prior to the inception of HRT [14]. It was also proposed to lower the dosage of estrogen with presumably the same results. There are postmenopausal women who do not tolerate some side effects of progesterone and prefer the single estrogen replacement therapy (ERT) despite its known potential carcinogenic risks. The effect of HRT on the uterus depends on the type of hormone, its dosage, and duration. The currently applied HRT (transdermal estradiol and micronized progesterone), recommended by the guidelines from the North American Menopause Society [14], elicits a wide range of histopathological changes of the endometrial structure observed on biopsies or endometrial aspirates (Vabra), often difficult to interpret and to differentiate from premalignant and even malignant changes. The latter are not common in HRT but may occur with ERT. In HRT, sometime atypical hyperplastic and neoplastic changes are associated with masquerading features such as stromal decidual reaction of various extents, occasionally even imitating gestational changes.

3.1 *Effects of ERT*

Effects of ERT (estrogen alone, unopposed by progesterone) on the uterus are positively related to the duration of exposure. They are ranging from weakly to markedly proliferative endometrium, similar to the proliferative phase of the normally cycling endometrium. There may be associated breakdown of the stroma due to small thrombi in the blood vessels, manifested clinically by postmenopausal vaginal bleeding, histologically often designated rather vaguely as "irregular proliferative endometrium". Prolonged use of this regimen may stimulate more proliferation of glands which appear crowded, lined by tall epithelial cells with large nuclei and displaying mitotic activity, as estrogens are mitogenic hormones. The crowded pattern is exaggerated by stromal breakdown.

The resulting pattern of "back to back" glands is suggestive of endometrial hyperplasia or neoplasia which has to be considered based on the presence of pseudo- and real epithelial stratification with loss of epithelial polarity, nuclear atypia, and atypical mitotic figures (Fig. 13a). Estrogen receptors are strongly positive (Fig. 13b). Crowding of otherwise benign fragmented glands or detached epithelial cells, due to the breakdown and disappearance of the intervening stroma, thrombosed blood vessels, and hemorrhagic areas are not uncommon. Other estrogenic effects on the endometrium is the formation of hyperplastic polyps growing on stalks with thick blood vessels, composed of hyperplastic glands that are more commonly not atypical and reversible. Squamoid metaplasia of endometrial glands, appearing as small nodules of polygonal eosinophilic epithelial cells, also called "morules" by analogy with (but not related to!) the early embryo, is also a prolonged

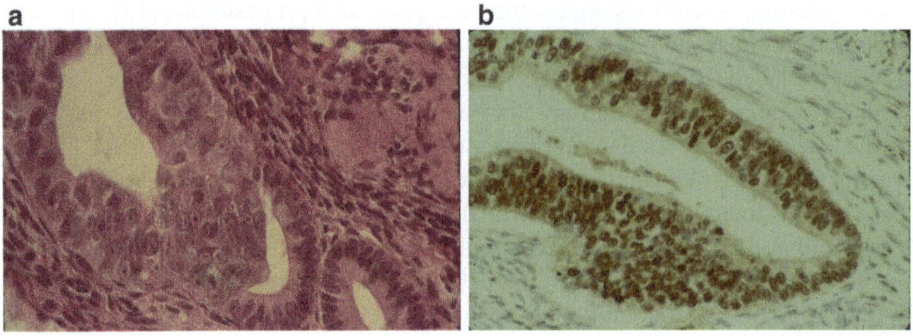

Fig. 13 (**a**) Effect of ERT on endometrium: atypical intraglandular hyperplasia with epithelial stratification, loss of polarity, nuclear atypia, mitotic activity. H&E ×100. (**b**) ERT effect on endometrium: Estrogen receptor stain strongly positive in atypical hyperplastic gland. Immunohistologic stain for ER ×100

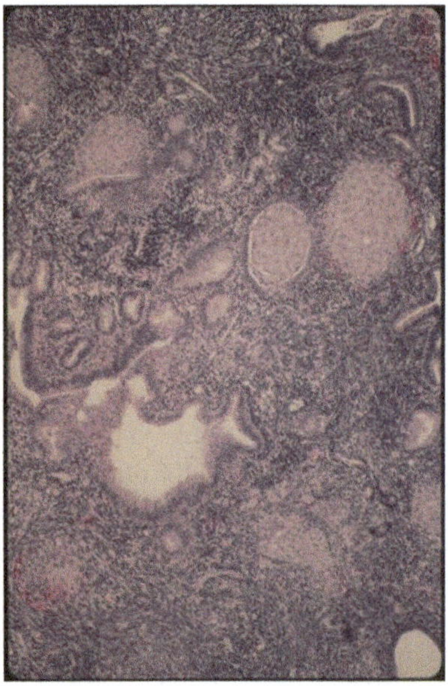

Fig. 14 ERT effect on endometrium: Atypical glandular hyperplasia with squamoid metaplasia (morules) H&E ×40

estrogen effect. These immature squamoid structures are usually metaplastic, therefore benign; they may fill the glands (Fig. 14) and appear as solid areas suggestive of, for the uninitiated, squamoid carcinoma especially when associated with atypical glandular hyperplasia. The endometrial stroma may respond to prolonged estrogen administration with accumulations of foamy macrophages with an abundant cytoplasm stuffed with lipid droplets representing deposits of steroid hormones. This finding in endometrial biopsies, although often associated with atypical hyperplasia or carcinoma, is in itself benign and may document a history of prior steroid hormone intake (Fig. 15).

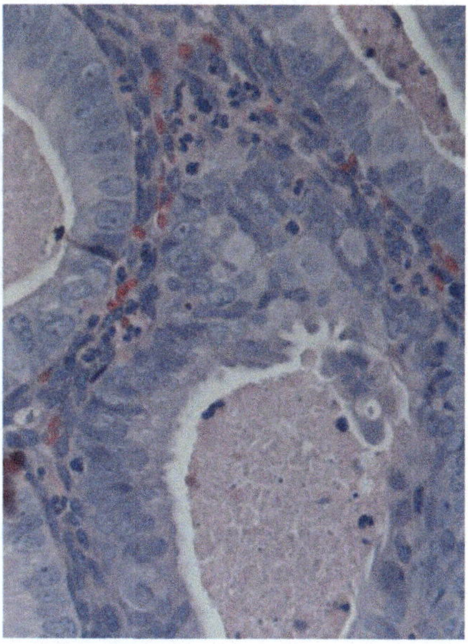

Fig. 15 ERT effect on endometrium: Atypical glandular hyperplasia and stromal foam cells H&E ×100

Prolonged ERT is also used in children with ambiguous genital development such as in Turner's syndrome at the time of puberty. The maternal hormones provide feminine development of Mullerian ducts during intrauterine life. At birth and in early childhood, the genital organs (uterus and fallopian tubes) are infantile and the absent ovaries are replaced by streak gonads. At the age of puberty, there is failure of menarche as the streak gonad failed to become an ovary due to the 45,XO karyotype lacking a second sex chromosome. No sex hormones are produced and the uterus remains infantile. Hormone replacement therapy is given to stimulate the uterine development and menarche at puberty.

As an example, a patient admitted to the emergency room with massive vaginal bleeding had been given ERT for 7 years (from the age of 12 to age 19). The uterus was found markedly enlarged containing polypous masses that histologically revealed an endometrioid adenocarcinoma for which hysterectomy was performed (Fig. 16a, b). Most, though not all, endometrial carcinomas developed during or after ERT are endometrioid (type I), strongly hormone receptor positive carcinomas with a rather favorable prognosis, as compared to the nonendometrioid (type II) seen less often in mostly older women, not treated with estrogens [15].

The effect of ERT after menopause on the myometrium is to stimulate, by receptor-binding to the myometrial tissue, the proliferation of myometrial tissue that may result in proliferating leiomyomas. Involution of the uterus and atrophy of the endometrium will take place after the cessation of hormone stimulation and/or exhaustion of hormone receptors.

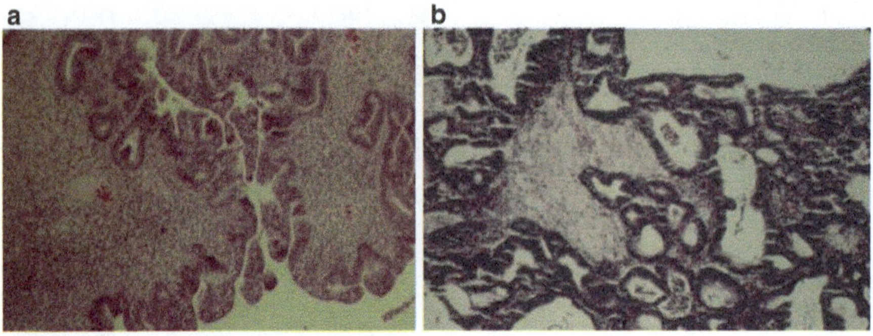

Fig. 16 (**a**) Effect of 7-year ERT duration on endometrial biopsy of a 19-year-old patient with Turner syndrome: well-differentiated adenocarcinoma, endometrioid type. H&E ×100. (**b**) Same patient, section of hysterectomy specimen: adenocarcinoma, endometrioid type H&E ×100

Table 2 Endometrial histology in HRT

Glands	Proliferative, weakly or as in early, mid or late proliferative phase
	Hyperplastic, without or with atypia, crowded, polypoid
	Secretory, early, mid or late
	Mixed proliferative and secretory
	Metaplasia: tubal (ciliated), squamoid (morules), mucinous, papillary
Stroma	Edematous
	Decidual reaction
	Breakdown as in menstrual shedding, hemorrhagic
Blood vessels	Spiral, thickened or thin
	Angiectasis, thrombosis
Any combination of the above	

3.2 *Effects of Combined HRT*

Effects of combined HRT on the uterus include a wide spectrum of structural changes (Table 2). Various combinations of proliferative and secretory patterns may be observed as a result of estrogenic and progesterone simultaneous stimulation: weakly to intensely proliferative glands and/or secretory glands with sub- and supranuclear secretory vacuoles and/or intraluminal secretion, consistent with various stages of glandular secretion. Associated secretory stromal changes range from edema to decidual reaction and compact decidualization analogous to gestational endometrium. The blood vessels range from thin and straight to thick and coiled similar to spiral arterioles seen in natural midsecretory endometrium. The overall histologic pattern may appear confusing when compared to the natural cyclic dating of the endometrium. Associated abnormal, though benign, histologic structures can include tubal (ciliated), eosinophilic, mucinous, or papillary metaplasia presenting an irregular pattern that especially when combined with glandular crowding may appear suspicious for neoplasm (Fig. 17). Pseudomenstrual changes consisting of vascular fibrinoid thrombosis, stromal breakdown, apoptosis, cellular debris with "nuclear dust," stromal polymorphonuclear leukocytic infiltrates may occur at the iatrogenic withdrawal of hormones, in an analogous way to menstrual endometrial shedding. With the currently combined HRT recommended by the guidelines of the North American Menopause Society, transdermal estradiol and micronized progesterone [14] a commonly seen histological pattern is that of proliferative glands and secretory-type glands resulting from the simultaneous intake of estrogen and progesterone (Fig.18a, b). Coexisting proliferative glands with decidualized stroma reflect the obviously iatrogenic predominant effect of progesterone therapy, simultaneous with a moderate estrogen effect (Fig. 19a, b). Predominant estrogen effect may elicit benign tubal (ciliated) metaplasia (Fig. 20a) and tubal metaplasia associated with glandular atypia (Fig. 20b) as well as squamoid metaplasia, as previously shown (Fig. 14). Predominant progesterone effect may show a late secretory-type endometrium, with stromal breakdown somehow reminiscent of premenstrual changes (Fig. 21) or decidualized stroma with inactive epithelium, reminiscent of gestational epithelium (Fig. 22). Prolonged therapy with combined HRT in postmenopausal women may eventually result in inactive endometrium with straight nonproliferating and nonsecreting glands and dense stroma (Fig. 23). This finding can occasionally be associated with functional and/or hyperplastic changes.

It is presumed that neoplastic changes are prevented by adding progesterone to estrogen therapy. This is however not always the case. Endometrial cystic glandular hyperplasia and irregularly proliferative glands are a relatively common finding (Fig. 24). Atypical endometrial hyperplasia (Fig. 14) and endometrial carcinoma (Fig. 25) are occasionally seen in postmenopausal women receiving combined HRT

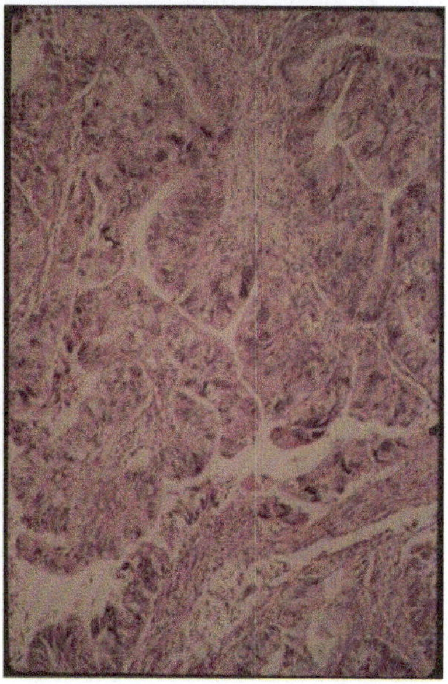

Fig. 17 Effect of combined HRT on endometrium: glandular crowding, mucinous, tubal, papillary metaplasia, nuclear atypia. H&E ×40

[16]. This can occur in some cases in which cyclic progesterone is administered for a shorter duration and in patients with risk factors such as obesity or estrogen-secreting ovarian tumors.

The effects of HRT on the endometrium are dose- and duration-dependent and reflect often in single samples puzzling features such as a combination of hormone depletion and hormone stimulation by both estrogens and progesterone.

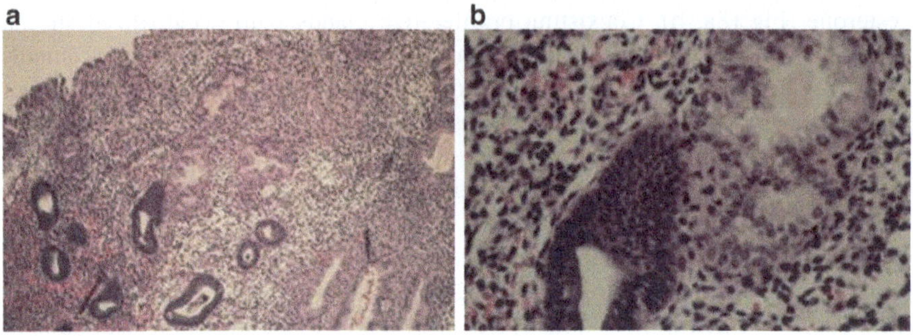

Fig. 18 Effect of combined HRT on endometrium: proliferative and secretory glands side by side. H&E ×40 (**a**) and 100 (**b**)

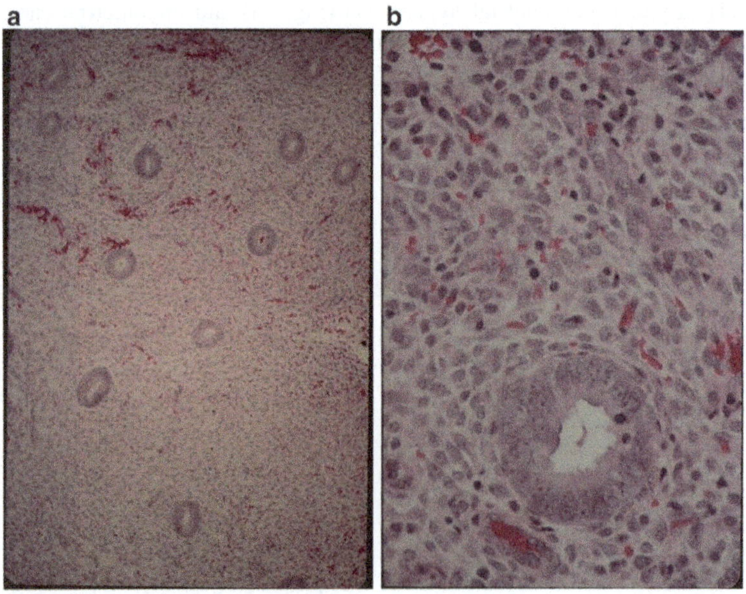

Fig. 19 (**a**) Effect of combined HRT on endometrium: stromal hyperplasia with decidual reaction and early proliferative-type glands. H&E ×25. (**b**) Effect of combined HRT on endometrium: proliferative gland with mitosis and decidualized stroma H&E ×100

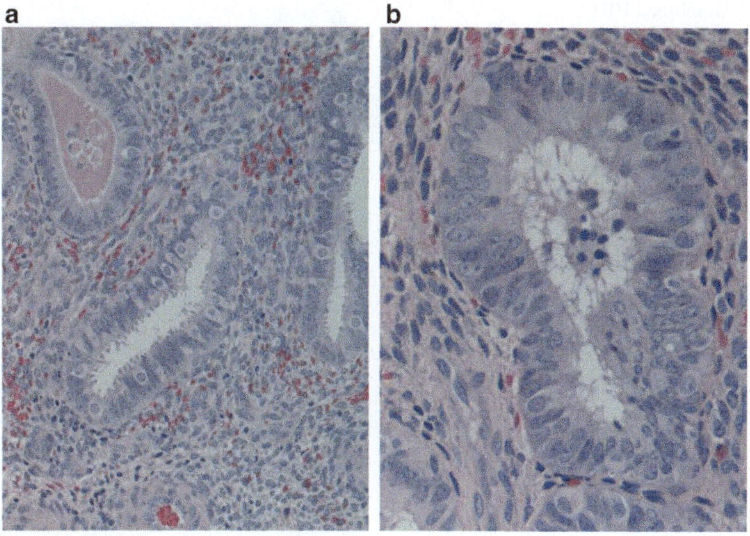

Fig. 20 (a) Combined HRT with predominant estrogen effect on endometrium: tubal metaplasia of glandular epithelium. H&E ×40. (b) Combined HRT with predominant estrogen effect on endometrium: Hyperplastic gland with tubal metaplasia and atypia. H&E ×100

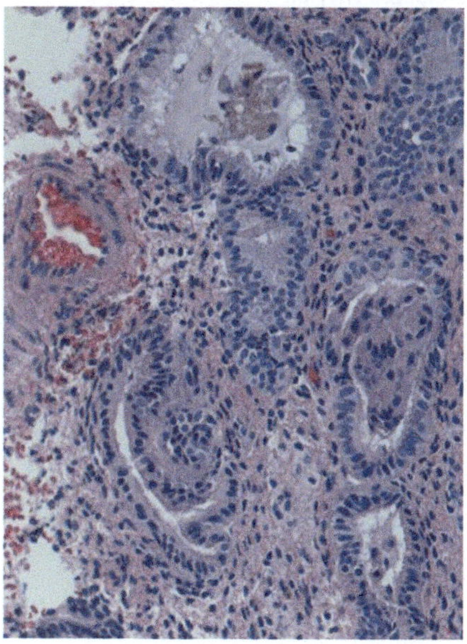

Fig. 21 Combined HRT with predominant progesterone effect on endometrium: secretory glands, early stromal breakdown. H&E ×40

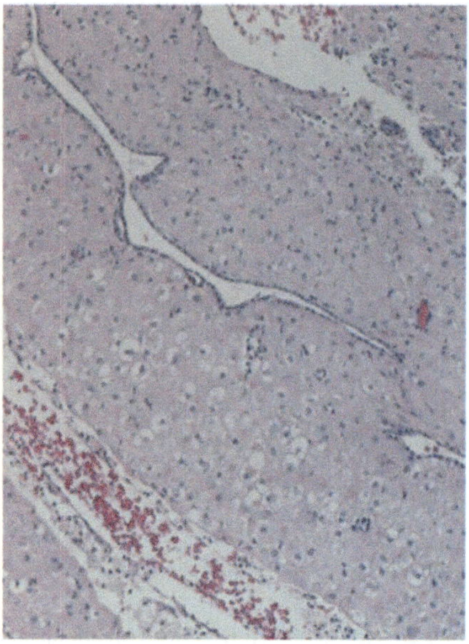

Fig. 22 Combined HRT with predominant progesterone effect on endometrium: decidualized stroma, inactive epithelium, similar to gestational endometrium. H&E ×25

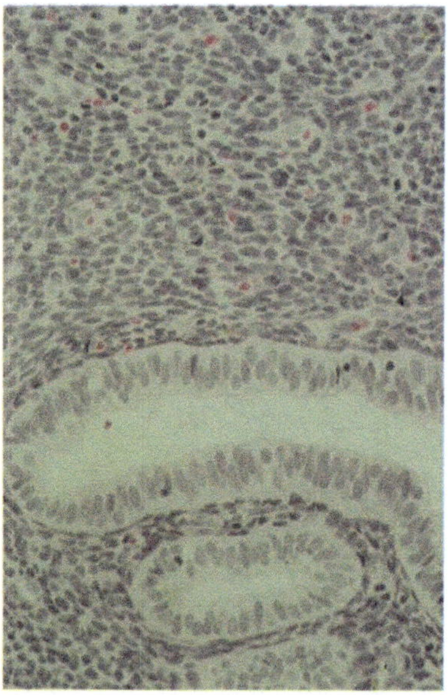

Fig. 23 Effect of prolonged HRT on endometrium: nonproliferative, nonsecretory inactive glands, dense stroma. H&E ×100

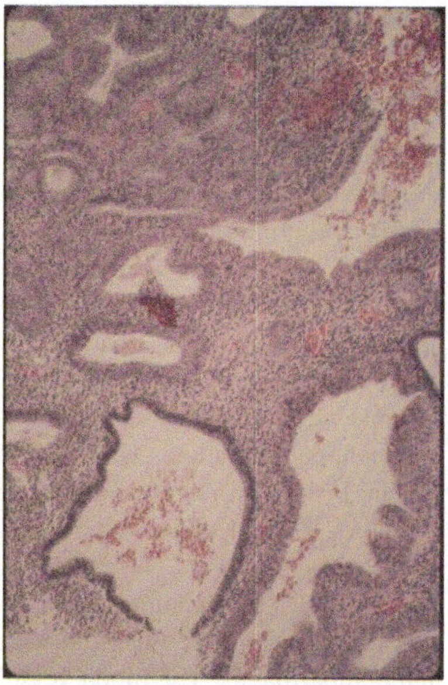

Fig. 24 Effect of combined HRT: Glandular cystic hyperplasia, focally atypical. H&E ×40

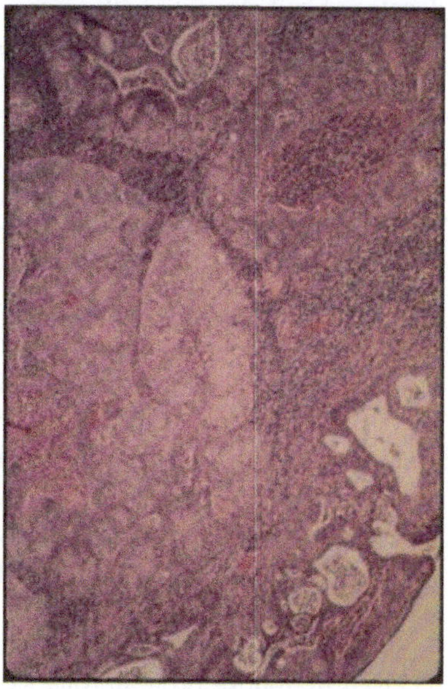

Fig. 25 Endometrial adenocarcinoma and glandular cystic hyperplasia in a 63-year-old patient receiving combined HRT for 7 years. H&E ×40

4 Effects of Antineoplastic Hormone Therapy

4.1 Progesterone Therapy

Progesterone therapy is often used in premenopausal patients diagnosed with endometrial hyperplasia based on its ability to inhibit DNA synthesis and to induce regression of abnormal endometrial proliferation. Medroxyprogesterone acetate (MPA) is the treatment of choice for endometrial glandular hyperplasia without atypia. High-dose progestins are also prescribed to reverse atypical glandular hyperplasia and as an adjuvant therapy for endometrial carcinoma especially for younger patients who want to preserve their uterus for reproductive purposes and for selected postmenopausal patients with contraindications for surgery [17].

The histologic response to progesterone therapy is mediated by progesterone receptors. The extent and intensity of the response correlates with the receptor level and distribution [18]. This therapy produces an arrest of glandular proliferation, epithelial secretory changes and stromal edema, and/or decidual reaction [19]. The endometrium appears quiescent with no or few mitoses in both glandular and stromal compartments. The blood vessels respond to progestins occasionally by thickening and coiling as in spiral arterioles. These changes however may be irregularly developed and alternate with areas of hyperplasia similar to those seen in the biopsies prior to therapy. Consecutive endometrial biopsies from patients diagnosed with endometrial hyperplasia treated with progesterone may show different histologic patterns with progressive decrease of hyperplasia especially in hyperplasia without atypia which is more responsive to this therapy.

The effect on the glandular epithelium is evident as secretory vacuoles, intraluminal secretion, stromal hyperplasia with decidual reaction and thickened arterioles, in various combinations. The volume of stromal tissue is increased compared to that of the glands. Cystic glands usually persist but may contain intraluminal secretion (Fig. 26a, b). The architectural changes due to prolonged and unopposed estrogenic stimulation in endometrial hyperplasia such as cystic dilation of the glands, irregular crowding, cribriforming, and outpouching tend to persist after progesterone therapy, while the epithelial lining of the glands appears more responsive: mitotic activity is decreased or absent, nuclei are regular and cells appear quiescent. In atypical endometrial glandular hyperplasia and in endometrial carcinoma adjuvant, progesterone therapy may fail to produce any effect or may produce only partial or focal change.

A 32-year-old patient with endometrial carcinoma refused surgical therapy and received high-dose progesterone (Megace) for 3 months. The endometrial biopsy showed partial secretory changes of the glands in this endometrioid adenocarcinoma (Fig. 27a). After subsequent 3 months of Megace therapy, the cribriform pattern persisted while the glands were secretory appearing quiescent, with no mitotic activity (Fig. 27b). Six months later, on the same therapy, the cribriform pattern persisted while the secretory changes became diffuse (Fig. 28). Hysterectomy was performed and histologic sections of the uterine wall displayed myometrial invasion

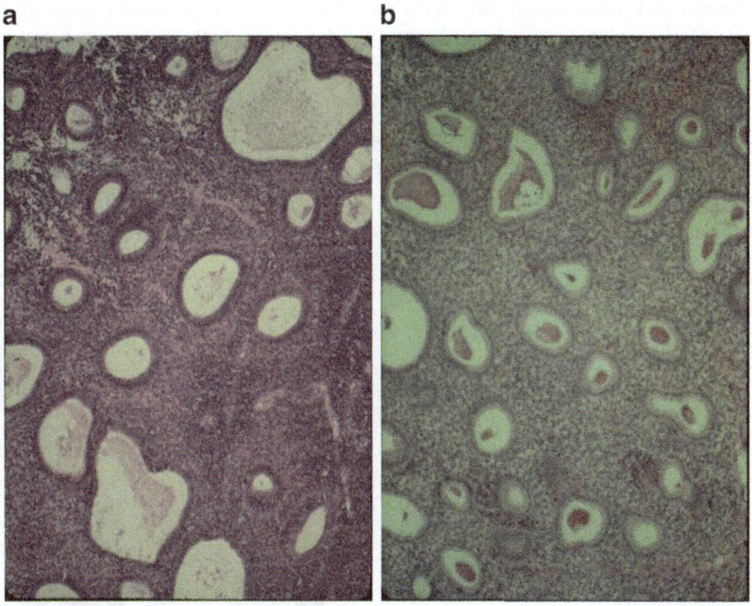

Fig. 26 (**a**) Nonatypical endometrial glandular-cystic hyperplasia, before HRT: proliferative epithelial lining of cysts. H&E ×40. (**b**) Same patient after 3 months of progesterone therapy: glandular cysts persist, lined by secretory epithelium, intraluminal secretion

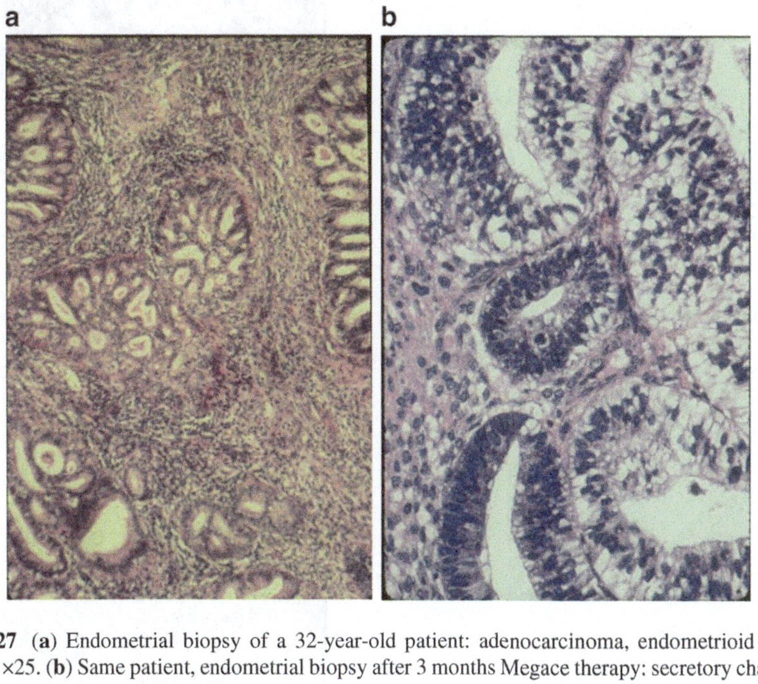

Fig. 27 (**a**) Endometrial biopsy of a 32-year-old patient: adenocarcinoma, endometrioid type. H&E ×25. (**b**) Same patient, endometrial biopsy after 3 months Megace therapy: secretory changes in neoplastic glands H&E ×100

by endometrioid adenocarcinoma with secretory glands ("secretory carcinoma" as it is called in some classifications) involving almost the full thickness of the uterine wall (Fig. 29).

In another 28-year-old obese patient diagnosed with endometrial adenocarcinoma, endometrioid type, the endometrial biopsy after 3 months of progesterone therapy showed on some histologic sections decidual tissue (Fig. 30), while on other sections cribriform glands with secretory changes were surrounded by a decidualized stroma (Fig. 31). On hysterectomy however, no invasive tumor was identified.

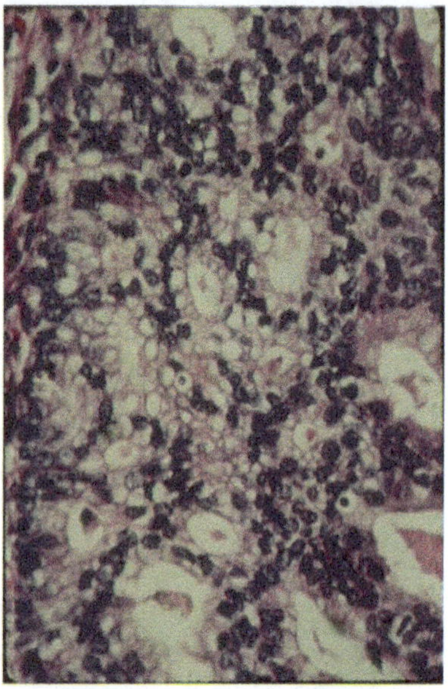

Fig. 28 Same patient after 6 months more of Megace therapy: endometrial adenocarcinoma with secretory changes. H&E ×100

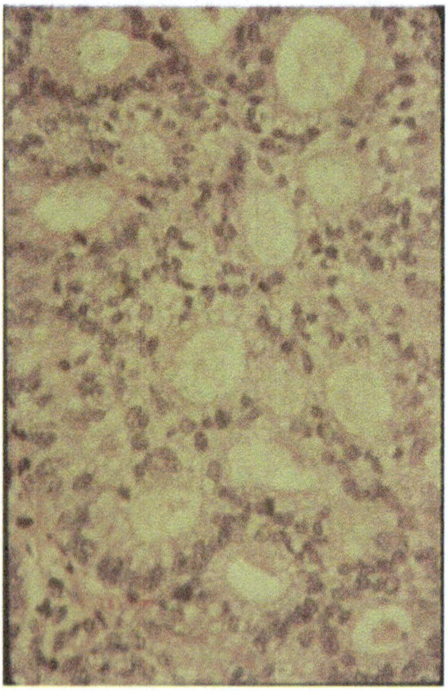

Fig. 29 Same patient after 2 months more of Megace therapy, section of hysterectomy specimen with diffuse myometrial invasion by adenocarcinoma displaying extensive secretory changes (secretory adenocarcinoma). H&E ×100

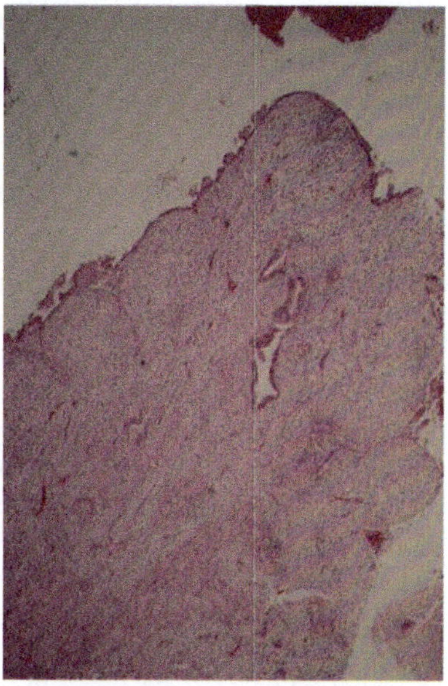

Fig. 30 Endometrial biopsy of a 28-year-old obese patient diagnosed with endometrial carcinoma, after 3 months Megace therapy: areas of diffuse stromal decidualizaton, some inactive glands. H&E ×25

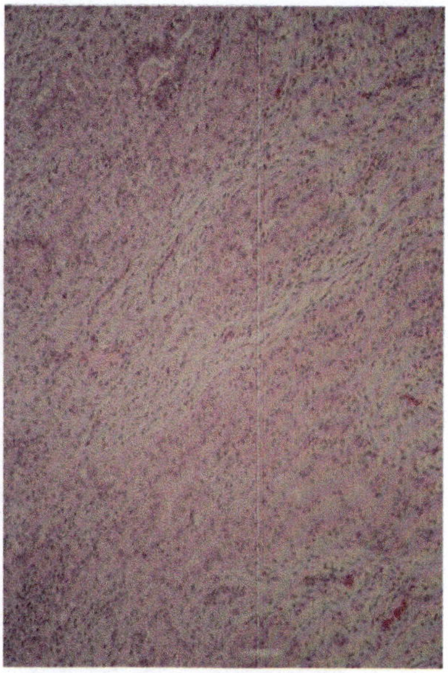

Fig. 31 Same biopsy (as in Fig. 30): adenocarcinoma, endometrioid type with secretory changes (secretory carcinoma) and stromal decidualization. H&E ×25

A "pseudopregnancy" histologic pattern (decidua, secretory glands) on endometrial biopsies therefore may be misleading by masquerading malignant changes.

Only careful and detailed examination of the hysterectomy specimen can rule out malignancy. Complete reversal of endometrial carcinoma by hormonal therapy is still a subject of debate, as is preservation of fertility in young women with endometrial neoplasia [20–23].

4.2 *Tamoxifen Therapy for Breast Cancer*

Tamoxifen is a nonsteroidal, synthetic triethylene estrogen derivative used successfully in the adjuvant therapy and prophylaxis of breast cancer. It binds to estrogen receptors in a manner similar to that of estradiol and induces binding of the tamoxifen/receptor complex to the nuclear DNA, resulting in a decrease of available unbound receptors. This explains the antiestrogenic effect on breast tissue. Its effect on the uterus is more complicated, being both antagonistic and agonistic to that of estrogens. The estrogen-agonist effect on the uterus is manifested by polypous proliferation with or without endometrial glandular hyperplasia ranging from cystic and nonatypical to atypical glands; areas of frank neoplasm in the polyps are occasionally present [24]. The stroma is different from that of endometrial hyperplastic polyps associated with a hyperestrogenic clinical background which display vascular and fibroblastic proliferation. Tamoxifen-related endometrial polyps usually display a mostly fibrotic stroma with few fibroblasts and often mucinous metaplasia of glands (Fig. 32a) as compared to nontreated endometrial polyps (Fig. 32b).

In the largest published histologic study of 700 cases of endometrial tissue from biopsies and hysterectomy specimens taken from patients treated with tamoxifen

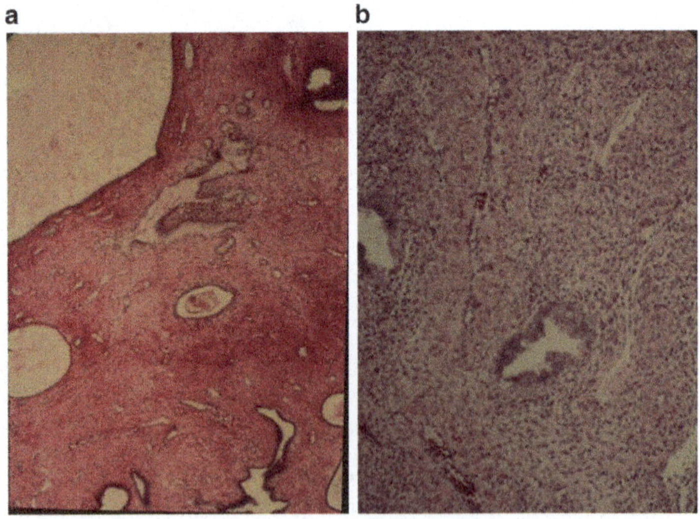

Fig. 32 (**a**) Patient treated with tamoxifen for breast cancer: endometrial polyp with cystic glands, mucinous metaplasia, and fibrous stroma. H&E ×25. (**b**) Endometrial polyp, no previous tamoxifen therapy: vascular thickening, endometrial inactive glands, and cellular stroma. H&E ×40

for breast cancer [25], the majority (64%) showed normal cycling or inactive endometrium. A significant number of patients (about 24%) had endometrial polyps composed of mostly inactive glands, some with mucinous metaplasia and some with benign hyperplastic changes, often cystically dilated (Fig. 31). Malignant changes were diagnosed in 4.7% of all cases, most often high-grade serous endometrial adenocarcinoma, interestingly enough not associated with atypical glandular hyperplasia as is the case in most estrogen-dependent endometrial carcinomas. Endometrial carcinoma was present in polyps displaying benign cystic changes and a fibrotic stroma (Fig. 33), with no background of glandular hyperplasia.

This is a different pattern from that of endometrial polyps involved by endometrioid carcinoma, usually associated with atypical hyperplasia. Only a third of the malignant endometrial cancers were endometrioid carcinomas (which overall are the majority of endometrial neoplasms), while two-thirds were poorly differentiated serous carcinomas (Fig. 34a, b). It seems therefore that both benign polyps and malignant endometrial neoplasms are histologically and biologically different from what is generally accepted as an estrogen-related endometrial neoplastic growth. This may be due possibly to different receptors: alpha-estradiol receptors in hyperestrogenic patients and beta-estradiol receptors in tamoxifen-treated patients. Also the proliferation of subendometrial nonglandular tissue which often mimics an endometrial thickening on ultrasound uterine images [26], raising suspicion of endometrial hyperplasia, is unrelated to Estradiol (E2 alpha) receptors. Multiple endometrial cancer reported cases associated with tamoxifen therapy were high grade neoplasms, including malignant mixed Muellerian tumors [27–29]. Increased

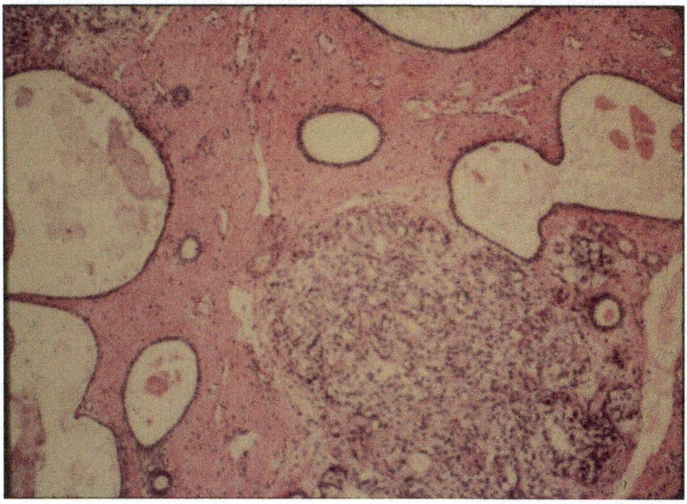

Fig. 33 Patient treated with tamoxifen for breast cancer: endometrial polyp with area of poorly differentiated adenocarcinoma and benign cystic glands in fibrotic stroma. H&E ×25

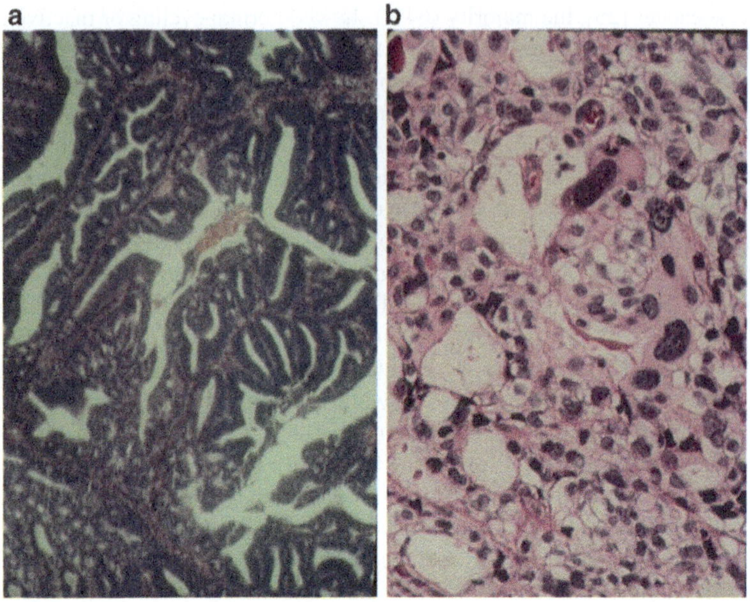

Fig. 34 (**a**) Patient treated with tamoxifen for breast cancer. Endometrial biopsy: adenocarcinoma, endometrioid type H&E ×40. (**b**) Patient treated with tamoxifen for breast cancer. Endometrial biopsy: high-grade serous carcinoma H&E ×100

aggressiveness of endometrial cancer has been associated with tamoxifen therapy due to recently identified genetic changes [30]. Tamoxifen-treated patients diagnosed with endometrial cancer were more common in older patients and in those who had a longer duration of therapy [25].

The estrogen-agonist effect of tamoxifen on the myometrium may include diffuse smooth muscle hyperplasia of the uterus (myohyperplasia), leiomyomata, adenomyosis with or without glandular hyperplasia. The size of the uterus may increase considerably in some cases reaching over 1200 g (Fig. 35a, b).

Despite the undesirable side effects of tamoxifen therapy on the uterus, it is now considered that the benefits (prevention of contralateral breast cancer recurrence, beneficial effect on cardiovascular and skeletal systems) exceed its deleterious side effects. It has been suggested that adding intrauterine levonogestrel to the tamoxifen therapy of breast cancer may prevent the risk of endometrial neoplasm [31]. Early detection of uterine malignancy is possible with careful surveillance including hysteroscopy, ultrasound examinations, and endometrial biopsies [32, 33] (Table 3).

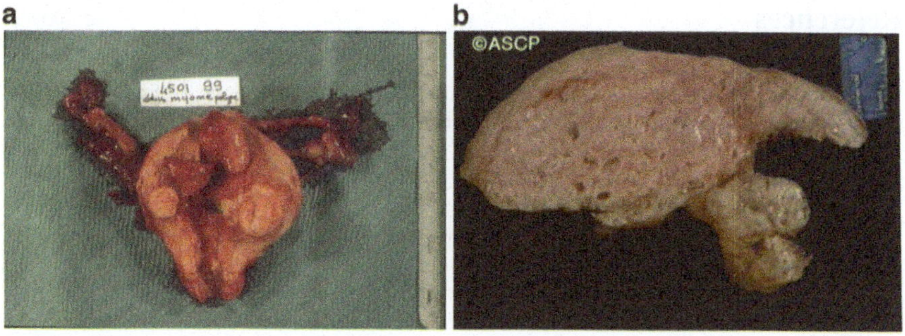

Fig. 35 (**a**) Patient treated with tamoxifen for breast cancer: massively enlarged uterus (980 g) with multiple leiomyomas and adenomyosis. (**b**) Patient treated with tamoxifen for breast cancer: massively enlarged uterus (1220 g) with diffuse adenomyosis and large endometrial polyp

Table 3 Tamoxifen therapy for breast cancer: effects on uterus

Endometrial cyclic changes
Inactive/atrophic endometrium
Metaplasia (mucinous most often)
Estrogen-agonist effects: leiomyoma, adenomyosis, myohyperplasia
Endometrial polyps with cystic and mostly non-atypical hyperplasia
Malignant tumors: endometrioid, serous high-grade carcinoma, malignant mixed Muellerian tumors (MMMT)

5 Conclusions

The diagnosis of uterine tissue, mostly of endometrial biopsies, from patients undergoing hormone therapy is often confusing and difficult to interpret [34]. This chapter presents a contemporary analysis meant to clarify the most commonly encountered issues, including oral contraception, ovarian stimulation, hormone replacement therapy, and antitumoral hormone therapy.

The histopathological patterns observed in the frequently taken endometrial biopsies from patients on hormone therapy encompass a wide variety of changes that cannot be sufficiently and adequately described in textbooks. They do not fit the classical descriptions of pathological noniatrogenic entities because of their diversity and the permanent change of therapeutic regimens, dosages as well as new concepts of therapy which represent challenges for both users and medical prescribers. A close clinical–pathological correlation and experience in gynecologic pathology is necessary for the interpretation of the often puzzling microscopic features of endometrial biopsies from hormonally treated patients.

References

1. Kase NG. The normal ovary part II: how steroid hormones work. In: Deligdisch L, Kase N, Cohen CJ, editors. Altchek's diagnosis and management of ovarian disorders. 3rd ed: Cambridge University Press; 2013. p. 37–63.
2. Kelley HW, Miles PA, Buster JE, Scragg W. Adenocarcinoma of the endometrium in women taking sequentially oral contraceptives. Obstet Gynecol. 1976;47:200–2.
3. Silverberg SG, Makovski EL. Endometrial carcinoma in young women taking oral contraceptive agents. Obstet Gynecol. 1975;46:503–6.
4. Mutter GL, Bergeron C, Deligdisch L, Ferenczy A, Glant M, Merino M, Williams AR, Blithe DL. The spectrum of endometrial pathology induced by progesterone receptor modulators. Mod Pathol. 2008;21:591–8.
5. Kathpalia SK, Kapoor K, Sharma A. Complications in pregnancies after in vitro fertilization and embryo transfer. Med J Armed Forces India. 2016;72:211–4.
6. Kushnir VA, Soloukis S, Sang-Moth-Vega MG, Albertini DF, Darmon SK, Deligdisch L, Barad DM, Gleicher N. Systemic inflammation and autoimmunity in women with chronic endometritis. Am J Reprod Immunol. 2016;75:672–7.
7. Minig L, Franchi D, Boveri S, Casadio C, Bocciolone L, Sideri M. Progestin intrauterine device and GnRH analogue for uterus-sparing treatment of endometrial precancers and well-differentiated early endometrial carcinoma in young women. Ann Oncol. 2011;22:643–9.
8. Deligdisch L, Hirschmann S, Altchek A. Pathologic changes in gonadotropin releasing hormone agonist analogue treated uterine leiomyomata. Fertil Steril. 1997;67:837–41.
9. Donnez J, Tatarchuk TF, Bouchard P, et al. Ullipristal acetate versus placebo for fibroid treatment before surgery. N Engl J Med. 2012;366:409–20.
10. Gusberg SB. Precursors of corpus carcinoma: estrogens and adenomatous hyperplasia. Am J Obstet Gynecol. 1974;54:905–27.
11. Kistner R. Alterations associated with estrogen-and estrogen-progestin combinations. In: The uterus. Baltimore MD: The Williams and Wilkins Co.; 1973, Monograph No 14, Chapter 12.
12. Kase NG. A clinical approach to post-menopausal hormone therapy. In: Altchek's diagnosis and management of ovarian disorders; 2013. p. 314–7. Chapter 20: Menopause.
13. Rossouw JE, Anderson GL, Prentice RL, et al. Risks and benefits of estrogen plus progestin in healthy postmenopausal women. JAMA. 2002;288:321–33.
14. The NAMS 2017 Hormone Therapy Position Statement Advisory Panel. The 2017 hormone therapy position statement of The North American Menopause Society. Menopause. 2017;24:728–53.
15. Deligdisch L, Kase NG, Bleiweiss IJ. Endometrial cancer in elderly women: a histologic and steroid receptor study. Gerontology. 2000;46:17–21.
16. Bereford SA, Weiss NS, Voigt LF, McKnight B. Risk of endometrial Cancer in relation to use of estrogen combined with cyclic progestogen therapy in post-menopausal women. Lancet. 1997;349:458–61.
17. Zaino RJ, Brady WE, Todd W, Leslie K, Fischer EG, Horowitz NS, Mannel RS, Walker JL, Ivanovic M, Duska LR. Histologic effects of medroxyprogesterone acetate on endometrial adenocarcinoma: a Gynecologic Oncology Group study. Int Gynecol Oncol. 2014;33:543–53.
18. Patell B, Figueroa S, Thakore S, Dahoud W, Bedalwy M, Messiano S. Role of nuclear progesterone receptor isoforms in uterine pathophysiology. Hum Reprod Update. 2014;21:155–73.
19. Randall TC, Kurman RJ. Progestin treatment of atypical hyperplasia and well differentiated carcinoma of the endometrium in women under age 40. Obstet Gynecol. 1997;90:434–40.
20. Falcone F, Laurelli G, Losito S, DiNapoli M, Granata V, Greggi S. Fertility preserving treatment with hysteroscopic resection followed by progestin therapy in young women with early endometrial cancer. J Gynecol Oncol. 2017;28(1):e2. https://doi.org/10.3802/jgo.2017.28.e2.
21. Inoue O, Hamatani T, Susumu N, Yamagami W, Ogawa S, Takemoto T, Hirasawa A, Banno K, Kuji N, Tanaka M, Aoki D. Factors affecting pregnancy in young women treated with

fertility-preserving therapy for well-differentiated endometrial cancer or atypical endometrial hyperplasia. Reprod Biol Endocrinol. 2016;14:2. https://doi.org/10.1186/s12958-015-0136-7.
22. van Gent MD, Nicolae Cristea AR, de Kroon CD, Osse EM, Kagie MJ, Trimbos JB, Hazelbag HM, Smit VT, Bosse T. Exploring morphologic and molecular aspects of endometrial cancer under progesterone treatment in the context of fertility preservation. Int J Gynecol Cancer. 2016;26(3):483–90. https://doi.org/10.1097/IGC.0000000000000629.
23. Mentrikovsky MJ, Shah AA, Hanley KZ, Atkins KA. Assessing endometrial hyperplasia and carcinoma treated with progestin therapy. Am J Clin Pathol. 2012;138:524–34.
24. Schlesinger C, Kamoi S, Ascher S, Kendell M, Lage JM, Silverberg SG. Endometrial polyps: a comparison study of patients receiving tamoxifen with two control groups. Int J Gynecol Pathol. 1998;17:302–11.
25. Deligdisch L, Kalir T, Cohen CJ, De Latour M, Le Bouedec G, Penault-Llorca F. Endometrial histopathology in 700 patients treated with tamoxifen for breast cancer. Gynecol Pathol. 2000;78:181–6. Selected for Breast Diseases: A Yearbook Quarterly 2001, publ. Mosby Yearbook Inc.
26. Dieudonne AS, Lambrechts D, Smeets D, Belmans A, Wildiers H, Paridaens R, Hyonil C, Timmerman D, Christiaens MR, Vergote I, Neven P. The rs 1800716 variant in CYP2D6 is associated with an increased double endometrial thickness in post-menopausal women on tamoxifen. Ann Oncol. 2014;25:90–5.
27. Magriples U, Naftolin F, Schwartz PE, Carcangiu M. High-grade endometrial carcinoma in tamoxifen-treated breast cancer patients J. Clin Oncol. 1993;11:485–90.
28. Clement PB, Oliva E, Young RH. Mullerian adenosarcoma of the uterine corpus associated with tamoxifen therapy: a report of six cases and a review of tamoxifen-associated lesions. Int J Gynecol Pathol. 1996;15:222–9.
29. Robinson DC, Bloss JD, Schiano MA. A retrospective study of tamoxifen and endometrial cancer in breast cancer patients. Gynecol Oncol. 1995;59:186–90.
30. Hrstka R, Podhorec J, Nenutil R, Sommerova L, Obacz J, Durech M, Faktor J, Bouchal P, Skoupilova H, Vojtesek B. Tamoxifen-dependent induction of AGR2 is associated with increased aggressiveness of endometrial cancer cells. Cancer Investig. 2017;35:313–24.
31. Gizzo S, Gangi S, Bertocco A, Noventa M, Fagherazzi S, Ancona E, Saccardi C, Patrelli TS, D'Antona D, Nardelli GB. Levonogestrel intrauterine system in adjuvant tamoxifen treatment: balance of breast risks and endometrial benefits-systematic review of literature. Reprod Sci. 2014;21:423–31.
32. Saccardi C, Gizzo S, Patrelli TS, Ancona E, Anis O, Di Gangi S, Vacillotto A, D'Antona D, Nardelli GN. Endometrial surveillance in tamoxifen users: role, timing and accuracy of hysteroscopic investigation: observational longitudinal cohort study. Endocr Relat Cancer. 2013;20:455–62.
33. Lee Y, Park YR, Kim HR, Lee JW. Event-free survival following early endometrial events in breast cancer patients treated with anti-hormonal therapy. A nationwide claims data study. Medicine (Baltimore). 2019;98:e13976.
34. Deligdisch L. Hormonal pathology of the endometrium. Mod Pathol. 2000;13:285–94.

Index

L. Deligdisch-Schor, A. Mareş Miceli (eds.), *Hormonal Pathology of the Uterus*, Advances in Experimental Medicine and Biology 1242,
https://doi.org/10.1007/978-3-030-38474-6

The manufacturer's authorised representative in the EU is Springer Nature Customer Service Centre GmbH, Europaplatz 3, 69115 Heidelberg, Germany. If you have any concerns regarding our products, please contact ProductSafety@springernature.com

Printed and bound by CPI Group (UK) Ltd, Croydon, CR0 4YY
30/07/2026
02181684-0003